FRIDGE LOVE

ORGANIZE YOUR REFRIGERATOR FOR
A HEALTHIER, HAPPIER LIFE—WITH 100 RECIPES

KRISTEN HONG

MARINER BOOKS
An Imprint of HarperCollins*Publishers*
Boston   New York

Photographs on pages ii, xi, xiv, xviii, 14, 83, 151, 153, 154, and 163 © 2022 by Jenn Bartell
Food photography © 2022 by Lauren Volo
Illustrations © 2022 by Amber Day

marinerbooks.com

Book design by Rita Sowins / Sowins Design

Library of Congress Cataloging-in-Publication Data has been applied for.
ISBN 978-0-358-43472-6 (POB)
ISBN 978-0-358-43547-1 (ebk)

Printed in Italy
RTL 10 9 8 7 6 5 4 3 2 1

FRIDGE LOVE

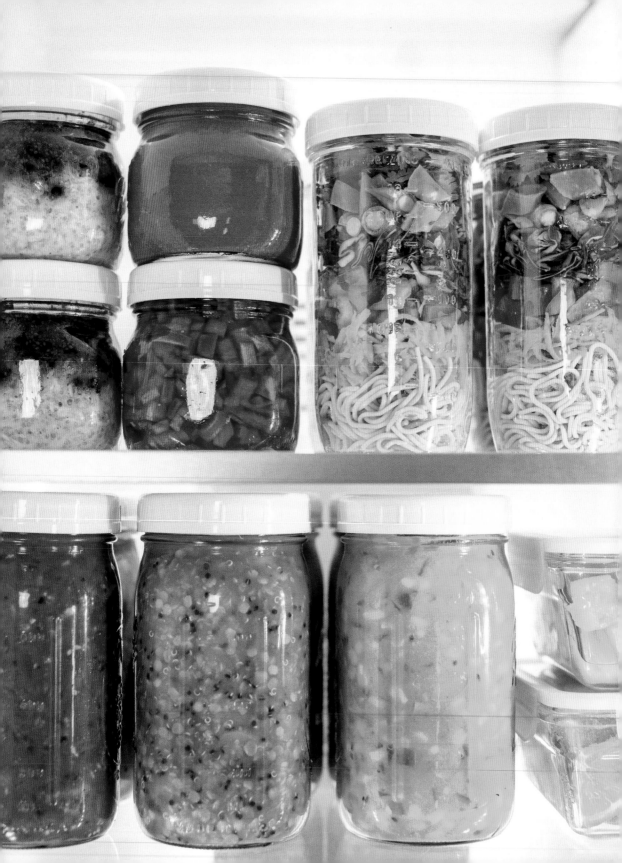

If you ever needed proof that amazing things can happen when you just keep trying, you're holding it in your hands.

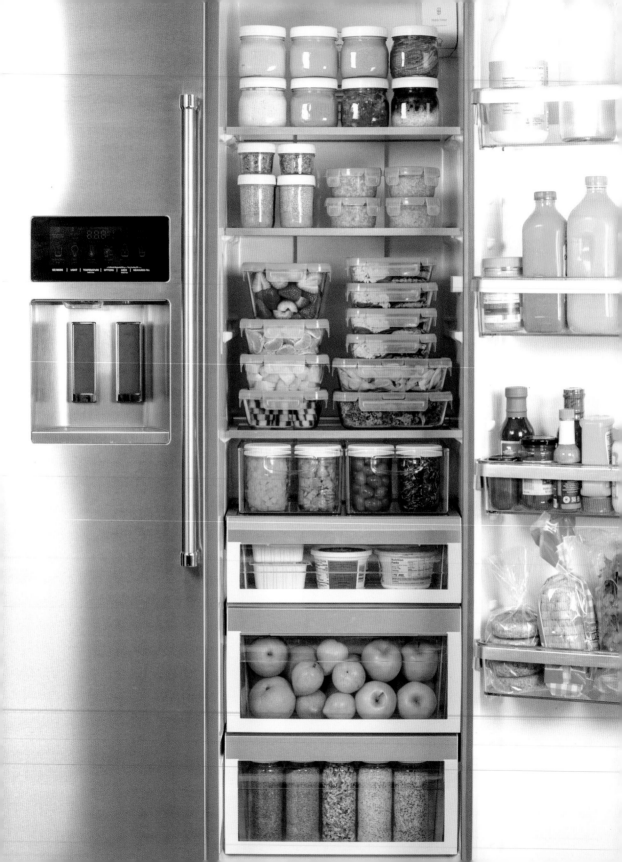

CONTENTS

INTRODUCTION

Just like a clean and organized desk increases your productivity at work, a clean and organized fridge will help you be more productive at adopting your healthy lifestyle, no matter what diet you follow (or don't follow!).

By now, we've collectively acknowledged the importance of practicing self-love. Usually that looks like morning yoga practice, meditation, and gratitude journals. And I think all of that is important. But now it's time to add a new form of self-love into the mix: taking the time to organize and stock your fridge to fuel your healthy lifestyle. I call this fridge love.

I dedicate time and effort to treating my fridge like a temple because it pays me back in good health, mental calmness, thriftiness, and a smaller carbon footprint on this earth. In short, it aligns me with my values. More than any other form of self-love I practice, making my fridge a top life priority has most helped me in living up to my potential. Every single day that I practice fridge love builds my confidence and resolve that I'm keeping my priorities straight. Fridge love is how I stay dedicated to my path living in what I lovingly call a "dietarily blended" family.

My fridge fuels me. And so I've created this resource for you, sharing everything I've learned about organization, fridge functionality, food storage, meal prepping, and other best practices. My goal for you is that after reading this book, you'll turn your fridge into your most powerful tool for your health! After all, what you put in your fridge inevitably ends up on your plate.

We'll work together to identify your own personal fridge objective, then I'll help you understand the basics of how your refrigerator works, present you with options for functional storage and organization strategies, share the ultimate produce and food shelf-life guide, and finally provide you with delicious recipes that will support your healthy fridge practice and personal goals (whether you're just here to get things organized or you're ready to make the leap into full weekly meal prepping).

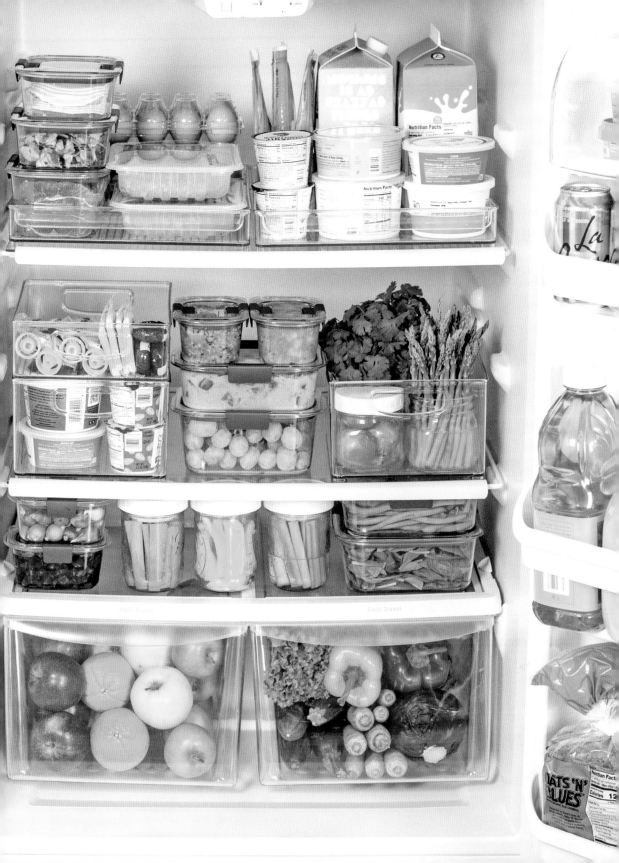

I've been made fun of on television for taking pictures of my fridge. A few years ago, one of my blog readers sent me a clip from her hometown Philadelphia news station.

They had done a segment that pretty much amounted to: "Look at these people wasting all their time posting pictures of their *fridges* on Instagram! How foolish are they?" Lots of smug laughing and comments along the lines of "Well, she certainly has too much time on her hands!"

Now, I've had to defend what I do over the years against rude emails, snarky comments, and purposefully vindictive reviews. It's all been part of this strange world of blogging.

Having it happen on TV was new for me.

But that lousy moment right there helped me to truly galvanize my worth and my mission. I started blogging and posting on Instagram to share beauty and inspiration from my own personal pain. Sharing what I'd learned, and posting weekly photos of my fridge, was the way I celebrated transforming my health. That's nothing to be ashamed of. And guess what? One hundred thousand friends on Instagram think so, too!

Then something funny happened . . .

That very same fridge pic that had been callously ridiculed on TV was featured in the *Wall Street Journal* in an article on organizing your fridge.

I'm not going to feign being humble on this one, guys—it felt pretty darn redeeming being interviewed for that story. And even more amazing when the editor asked to include the picture of my fridge. After I hung up with the reporter, I thought how glad I was that I never gave up on doing my thing. I moved past the haters, and popular culture caught up with me.

My Health Journey

There was a time, not really so long ago, when what was in my fridge was a complete and absolute afterthought.

I lived, breathed, and consumed fast food or shelf-stable processed foods, and ate out at restaurants all. the. time.

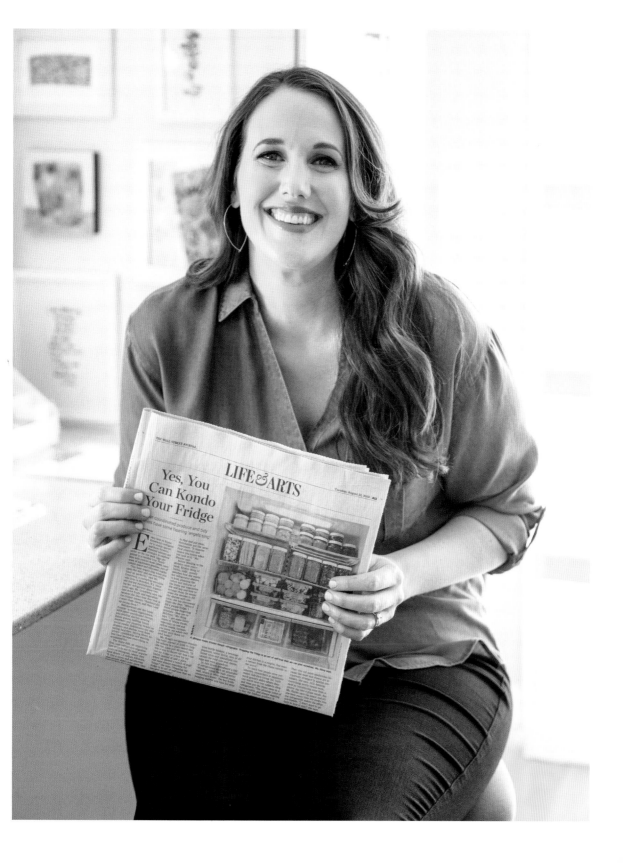

My fridge was merely the place my leftovers went to die.

For most of my adult life, the extent of my weekly "home cooking" had been Rice-A-Roni and Cup O'Noodles. My snacks came from bags, boxes, and cardboard canisters. Fresh fruits and veggies were garnishes on the foods I ate at restaurants—and I didn't particularly enjoy them.

It should come as no big surprise that I vacillated between being overweight or obese for much of that time. Even when I'd set my mind to "losing weight," that simply meant more processed food—stuffing my freezer with Lean Cuisines and counting calories. (I know, I know—the '90s called and they want their diet back!) I'd suffer for a few weeks to try to fit into a new outfit for a certain special occasion and then it was back to business as usual.

If you had taken a peek into my fridge at that time, you'd have found some booze, sodas, milk (for cereal), butter and eggs (you know, for the occasional boxed cake mix), and leftovers from the restaurants I frequented during the week.

I was completely squandering a gift of modern ingenuity—not to mention the money spent for the electricity required to house such paltry supplies. And I had absolutely no clue that what I kept in my fridge could have huge implications for my health.

THE CRASH DIET THAT REFUSED TO LEAVE

I finally started to pay some attention to my fridge when my youngest was six months old. With an 80-pound pregnancy weight gain that wouldn't budge, I was determined to head into my thirties putting my health first.

Becoming an example for my young family was a huge motivation. As luck would have it, the inspiration to make radical changes came from somewhere close to home.

Back in 2012, my mother came to visit. She looked like she had reverse-aged at least ten years, not to mention that she had lost a noticeable amount of weight. Nothing grabs your attention quicker than your mom looking younger than you!

The first thing I said when I picked her up from the airport was "What diet are you on?"

My mom told me that a few months earlier, my father had watched Dr. Joel Fuhrman on PBS and started following his high-nutrient eating plan called the Nutritarian diet. And since my dad did all the cooking, my mom followed along for the ride.

I immediately bought *Eat to Live*, Dr. Fuhrman's most popular book (over fifteen years later, it's still a bestseller). After reading it, I finally understood exactly how the "Standard American Diet" (SAD) had been impacting my health and weight over the years. And I realized that the only way to wrestle back my health was to embrace whole, natural foods.

I committed myself to following Dr. Fuhrman's six-week aggressive weight loss plan on the exact day my daughter turned six months old.

I had a still-breastfeeding infant, a toddler, and a husband who were all eating entirely different things, and I was the one doing all the cooking. Add to that a brand-new diet that was completely alien to me.

Needless to say, I was in for a crazy 42 days.

Now, I've graduated from law school and I've birthed two human beings, and I can tell you without a doubt that winging it through those first six weeks was one of the hardest things I've ever done.

But it worked.

Not only did I lose over 21 pounds without doing any exercise (besides leisurely walking), I finally experienced what it felt like to put my health first.

The craziest thing I'm about to tell you, which I know you won't believe until you experience it for yourself, is that the weight loss was the least meaningful change that happened for me during those first six weeks.

For the first time in my lifelong tortured existence with food, I felt peaceful and calm. My mind wasn't its usual loud chaotic mess: *When will I eat again? How can I sneak more food without my husband and kids noticing? Is the Taco Bell drive-through open this late?* All the mental energy I had wasted on food could now be applied to my goals. I was finally thriving—experiencing natural energy, mental focus, an elevated mood, and increased positivity.

I got hooked on those high-nutrient feels.

But getting yourself free from processed foods is, well, a process. We're all here right now because I didn't give up the struggle to convert what could have been a short-term diet into my forever lifestyle. What happened after those 42 days was years of falling off track, restarting, and failing again. My biggest obstacle was that I couldn't control my environment. My hubby

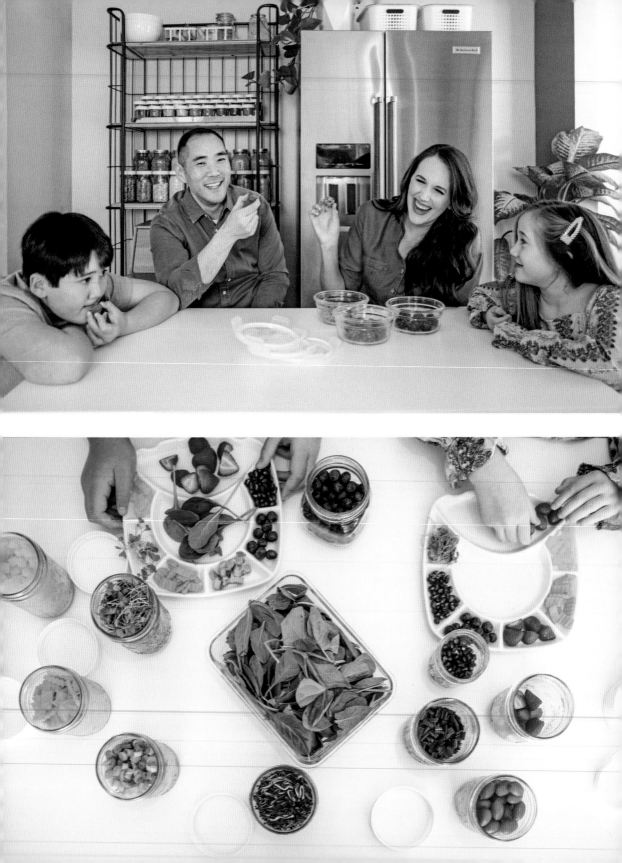

and kids were not going to be Nutritarians, so I had to live with those still-tempting SAD foods. So, after about 3 years of trying and struggling, I got strategic. I couldn't control my whole environment, but I could certainly control parts of it. I couldn't completely convert my family, but I could ask them to make reasonable concessions.

And that's how the fridge takeover, er, I mean, reorganization started.

I decided that if I was the one doing all the cooking, then my health and well-being had to be first priority. If I was the one eating the healthiest foods in the family, then those foods should take center stage in our lives.

I became resolutely unapologetic about pursuing my health goals.

As a mom, I set the tone for my family's health. My hubby and kids aren't Nutritarian vegans like I am. They still eat meat, dairy, sugar, and processed foods, but those foods are minimized in our home and my foods are maximized. They are living in a high-nutrient-centric household.

After years at this game, my kids eat raw and cooked veggies by habit. And I can tell you with 1,000 percent certainty that they eat waaaay more whole fruits and veggies than average kids their age. Our family standards have changed for the better. And that's because I was determined to make my healthy lifestyle stick and work within our family. Now my lifestyle and my example have set the tone for everyone else. I'm the linchpin of health for my family, and if you're a mom, you will be, too!

I started out by seeking time-saving strategies so I could cook two sets of meals during the week: one for my family and one for me. I had to make sure my food was easy to see and grab in the fridge so that once I had their dinner close to being done, I could pull out my ingredients and quickly assemble a Nutritarian meal. Then I took it a step further, because I was sick of cooking two meals every night and feeling like my food was always the afterthought. I started taking a few hours on the weekend to make meals I could heat up for myself during the week, while I cooked on-demand for my family.

After so many years, it has been proven to me that the time I dedicate to refrigerator organization and meal prepping sets us all up for success, week after week. Even though we're all on different dietary paths, we can come together around the food we love in a more relaxed and grateful way.

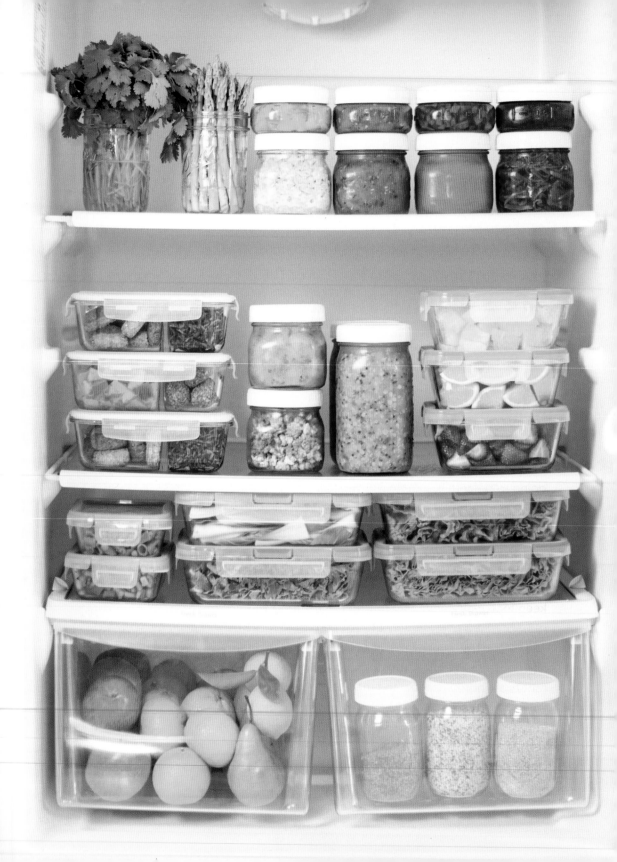

LET'S ANSWER ALL THE QUESTIONS

What if everything you needed to know about transforming and stocking your fridge was in one place? No matter if you're looking to go all in on high-nutrient living or you just want to become more intentional in how you set up and use your fridge to support the healthy lifestyle of your dreams, this resource is going to guide the way.

Your fridge is about to level up. When you share pics of your prepped fridges on Instagram, you get asked a whole lot of questions:

"How long will all this prepped food last you?"

"Do you prewash all your produce?"

"How many people eat from this fridge?"

"Do you have a second fridge where you keep all the normal things?"

"Won't your greens wilt and things get soggy and go bad?"

"Do you recommend glass or plastic storage containers?"

"Do you store chopped veggies in water or with paper towels or napkins?"

And that's just the tip of the iceberg lettuce. In this book, you'll get every tip, trick, and scientific tidbit of information you need in order to never feel like you're wasting your food budget ever again. Just think: Fridge waste doesn't live here anymore!

After reading this guide and putting the information into practice, you're going to be getting the maximum output from your fridge. You're going to know that a whole red cabbage keeps for up to 4 weeks in the fridge, whereas chopped red cabbage will keep for just 3 weeks—and if you thinly slice that chopped red cabbage, it will lose its freshness faster still. Then you're going to learn what to *do* with that red cabbage, like using it in your weekly in-fridge salad bar and in delicious, easy-to-make, high-nutrient recipes that keep for a week or longer in your fridge! I have no place in my life for twenty-plus-item ingredient lists—and I have a sneaking suspicion you don't, either.

I'm going to show you how to transform your current fridge (that's right—no running out to get a new fridge required) into the number one most important tool for your health. You're going to be locked, loaded, and ready to make lasting changes to your health. And it's going to be colorful, fun, and easy.

So let's make change happen together!

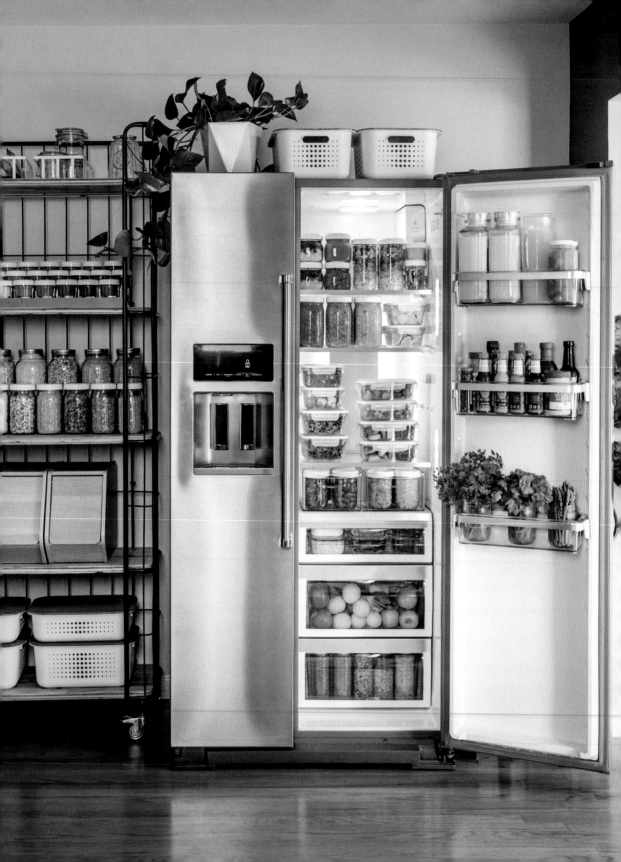

Part 1

PRACTICING FRIDGE LOVE

This book is your guide to getting every last drop of productivity, goodness, and nourishment from your fridge, and my hope is that you'll return to it again and again. I'm inviting you to join me in practicing fridge love, a new form of self-love—one where your time, intention, and health coalesce to make life easier for you and your family.

The way you practice fridge love is to:

- Appreciate that modern refrigeration is a gift.
- Love the fridge you're lucky enough to have right now.
- Learn to use your fridge to its fullest potential to fuel your health.
- Make peace with getting better at this with time.

You're going to come out of reading this book armed with the information, techniques, and recipes you need to practice fridge love in your own kitchen. This is a knowledge transfer of everything I've learned over years of prepping my fridge. I know this is life-changing stuff because I've seen it happen with so many readers who've shared their fridges with me over the years.

So let's start with the first step. It's an easy one, too. All you have to do is take a moment to remember something you've likely forgotten or maybe never even stopped to consider in the first place.

Recognizing the Gift

Modern refrigeration changed the game for humanity.

To truly start to care about the gift you have right now, we have to take a moment to remember just how bad we had it. Because truthfully, guys, when we complain about how "hard" it is to eat healthy, we sound like the most entitled, bratty bunch of ungrateful snobs ever. Consider this an intervention.

We stand in a moment in human history where we can habitually enjoy the healthiest foods possible. We have the infrastructure and the tech to make that miracle happen. Not all humans on this planet have access to the modern food system, so if you're reading these words right now, know that you're unquestionably one of the lucky ones.

None of this is to say that it's not hard to eat healthy. Even in our modern lives, there are plenty of barriers to accessing fresh, healthy foods. This can take the form of not having enough time or money to cook healthy meals or a lack of proximity to healthy food retailers. But the simple fact that you own or have reliable daily access to a refrigerator already sets you apart on this earth. It makes the pursuit of food easier, and it stretches out what food you do have.

And this is a gift.

It's a gift I want you to appreciate.

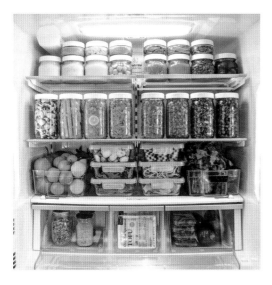
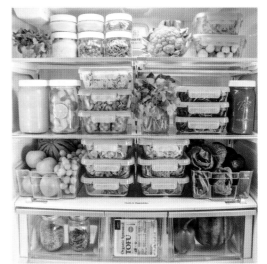
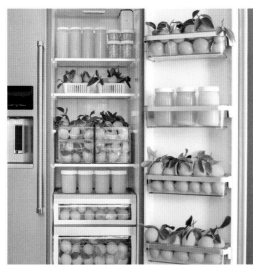
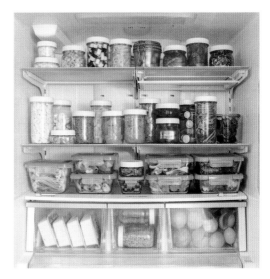
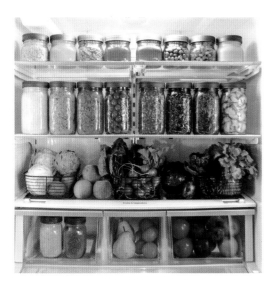
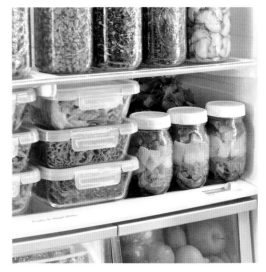

It's a gift I want you to utilize.

No matter your social or economic status or your life situation, you can take this gift (your fridge—whatever fridge you have, whether meager or splendid) and have it better serve your health right now.

So let's get calibrated. Let's take a minute to remember how things were so we can better appreciate how good we have it right now. It's the first step toward gratitude for one of the modern luxuries that we absolutely take for granted.

OUR QUEST FOR FOOD PRESERVATION

Modern refrigeration is only about 150 years old; before then, drying, smoking, salting, slathering foods with honey (and later sugar), pickling, and fermenting were the predominant ways to preserve food for future use (and of course, people still employ these techniques today).

Before refrigeration, so much of what you could do to preserve your food, and the ease of that preservation, was based on your location. If you were lucky enough to live in a temperate climate, during the winter you could use a root cellar and the snow itself to safely pack and preserve meat and other highly perishable foods. But if you lived in a humid environment, preserving food by drying it was a difficult and labor-intensive task. Things in the food preservation department were particularly tough in hotter, more humid climates. (I was born and raised in Miami, Florida, so I can both corroborate and appreciate this truth.)

The lifestyles we enjoy today were made possible by a quantum leap in food preservation technology. Since storage temperature is the number one reason food spoils, we had to figure out how to re-create cold environments in our cities and homes.

THE ICEBOX COMETH

Prehistoric man harnessed the power of heat and fire over one million years ago, but when did humanity begin to harness the power of cold? It all started with the pursuit of a good glass of wine. Well, in this case, a cool glass of wine.

Unsurprisingly, the first icehouses and ancient forays into cooling were in desert civilizations, where getting your hands on some chilled wine or even a cool breeze on a stifling day was largely reserved for royalty and only the wealthiest citizens. (Yes, that means that even a fifteen-year-old fridge with a ding in the door and a missing handle—a fridge that may be similar to the one sitting in your kitchen right now—is indeed fit for a king!)

Ever wonder how Egyptian pharaohs imbibed their wine? Think hand-cooled. After sunset, teams of slaves would haul up large terra-cotta wine vats from underground cellars, then spend the night sprinkling the vats with water and, if there wasn't a sufficient breeze, fanning them. Just think of *that* the next time you enjoy a chilled rosé on a sultry night.

In ancient Persia, it wasn't until the fifth century BCE that common people could also enjoy cool drinks and iced desserts. This was thanks in part to the region's unique climate and geography—inherently dry with cool nighttime temperatures—which made it possible to harvest natural ice from the mountains in the winter and store it in innovative ice huts called *yakhchals*.

As time pressed on, so did the quest to bring cold to the masses and to the climates that needed it most. By the early 1800s, American businessmen were jumping into the burgeoning—and volatile—natural ice business, harvesting ice that formed naturally in the winter on the lakes and rivers in New England and transporting it by ship to hotter locales. With lots of trial and error involved, lost profits abounded until a reliable network was developed to handle a literally melting commodity. Eventually, the American ice trade stretched to Europe, the Caribbean, and as far away as India.

Households and businesses would contract with ice companies for steady deliveries of large blocks of ice. After delivery, the ice could be stored in an icebox, a large wooden cabinet with two compartments: one for ice and the other for food. Air would circulate through vents from the ice compartment into the food compartment, keeping it cool. In a well-insulated unit, an ice block could last for five to seven days. Some iceboxes were downright beautiful—think of a china cabinet, but for ice and food (just search "McCray iceboxes" to see what I mean). By the 1830s, American households were accustomed to keeping dairy products and other perishable foods in an icebox. For the first time ever, people could actually save their leftovers!

In the nineteenth century, naturally sourced American northeastern ice was the most prized ice in the world. Consumers prized natural products as being inherently pure and clean and distrusted mechanically produced goods. But by the 1880s, the United States had developed a pretty insatiable domestic ice habit, consuming more than five million tons of ice annually. As demand outpaced supply, natural ice harvesters began to cut corners—selecting water sources that were nearer to population centers and prone to contaminated runoff.

After a few decades of disease outbreaks caused by pollutants in natural-ice water sources, the world was primed for artificial ice. New steam-powered ice factories gained traction and marketed their product as the safer alternative, since they boiled their water before freezing it—effectively killing pathogens. While artificial ice was undoubtedly more expensive, the deliveries were more consistent, as manufacturers were no longer dependent on harvesting only in the winter months. Ice was now available year-round, and in the end, consumers valued that reliability over the increased cost.

But the icebox, humanity's first foray into a household food preservation system, wasn't without its limitations and inconveniences. The earliest wooden iceboxes were quite large—like, *they-could-swallow-your-fridge-whole* large—but much of their volume was dedicated to housing the ice, so they had little storage space for actual food. There were other problems as well. When food was kept too close to the ice compartment, it caused food damage in the form of freezer burn. Also, the cold produced inside was a wet type of cold that wasn't ideal for many types of food. The temperature of a well-constructed icebox never reached below the mid-forties Fahrenheit (modern refrigerators run in the mid- to high thirties), and frequent opening of the icebox doors led to heat getting inside and the ice melting too fast.

There was also the issue of runoff. Depending on the model, the water from the melting ice would either be carried away by drainage pipes or collected in a drip tray that the homeowner would have to remember to dump out periodically. And if you think cleaning your fridge is a drag, do yourself a favor and read how to clean an icebox. It was a time-intensive process and had to be done weekly to prevent odors permeating the wooden container.

Still, for all their manifold drawbacks, iceboxes were superior to other common forms of food preservation at the time, especially for storing fresh items like milk, eggs, and meat. It was the first significant step toward preserving fresh foods and cutting food waste. The next step? Getting the ice out of the icebox for household cold that didn't require so much maintenance.

REFRIGERATORS RISING

Just as artificial ice would dethrone natural ice in consumer consciousness, manufacturers had to convince American households that mechanical cold storage was safer and better than the icebox.

Many of us know how the very first computers were so big, they filled up a large room. Well, fridges started out much the same way. Refrigerators were huge, hulking, dangerous machines that required trained technicians, contained chemicals known to be poisonous, and tended to spontaneously explode.

It wasn't a very encouraging beginning—but it was a beginning.

It would take over one hundred years of experimenting to find the right combination of gas and machinery. Starting in the early nineteenth century, the key to unlocking refrigeration was understanding how gases heated, compressed, and expanded.

The mysterious gas that makes our fridges run is known by the benign and even friendly sounding term "refrigerant," but the first gases used as refrigerants were anything but. The first two refrigerants used were ether and ammonia, both of which are highly flammable. Then came forays into using sulfur dioxide and carbon dioxide, precisely because they weren't flammable, but then toxic leaks were a problem. By 1873, a clear refrigerant-machinery-combo winner emerged: the ammonia compression fridge model. Now the size of the fridge had shrunk to the size of a room. Although the technology was still dangerous, as explosions continued to happen, it was embraced by commercial food and ice companies around the world, which were willing to handle the risk if it meant less inventory loss.

Emerging at the turn of the twentieth century, early home refrigeration history was a tangle of competing mechanical designs. The first home refrigerators required lots of space (the machinery was often housed in the basement, with a cold box in the kitchen) and lots of service calls. Unsurprisingly, the earliest home fridges were marketed to wealthy households, since they cost more than a Model T car.

It wasn't until 1927, with the release of General Electric's "Monitor Top" refrigerator, that modern refrigeration for the masses was born. Finally, manufacturing, engineering, and refrigerant technologies had matured to the point where the leaks, fires, and noise of the previous century's commercial fridges were a thing of the past. The compressor motors were small and powerful enough to cycle refrigerants, while also requiring less energy to run. And thanks to efficient assembly lines, middle-class families could enjoy the technology, too.

Every decade, the price of refrigerators fell and sales climbed, even during the Great Depression. Refrigerators were such an obvious upgrade to iceboxes that consumers couldn't resist buying one once the price was right. Predictably, modern refrigeration had a likely bedfellow in the burgeoning electricity industry. Electric utilities actually sold refrigerators directly to customers at a discount, making the long play that they'd make up the lost initial profit over years of increased energy use.

In the 1930s, new standard features began to develop, like adjustable shelves, better temperature controls, slide-out drawers, ice trays, automatic lights, and the first high-humidity drawers for fruits and veggies. By the end of the decade, the percentage of American households with a fridge had ballooned from 8 to 44.

After World War II, refrigerators got a key upgrade: frost-free technology. The old-school models accumulated frost around the refrigerant pipes, so you needed to turn the unit off and remove the ice by hand, being sure not to puncture the pipes in the process. In 1958, Frigidaire invented a way to use the heat generated by the compressor motor to automatically defrost the coils with every cycle.

Advances made after the marquee frost-free fridges have been largely aesthetic, and that's why we're going to end our introductory fridge history lesson here.

Repeat After Me: Any Working Fridge Works

"The basic difference in refrigerators has always been between those targeted at people from different economic groups."

—JONATHAN REES, AUTHOR OF *REFRIGERATOR*

Fridge technology—meaning the actual engineering—has changed very little over the past sixty years. Yes, individual components have improved and migrated to different areas of the fridge frame, better thermometers and more airflow spigots have sprouted up in pricier models, but the real changes have been to size, color, and configuration (side-by-side, French door, etc.).

As of the data available in 2015, you can expect a fridge to last you an average of between fourteen and seventeen years. It's only natural, then, that over 20 percent of homes in the US have a second fridge. When your old fridge never really stops working but you're ready for an upgrade, it makes sense to plop the old one in the garage or basement and instantly double your cold space. But it's not surprising that fridge longevity has presented a real problem for manufacturers wanting to drive sales.

Fridge manufacturers took a page from the auto industry. After all, how do you get people to buy or lease a new car every three or four years? You offer more bells and whistles, and you tie that car into their personal class identity. The fridge, like the car, becomes an object that signifies a person's economic status to others.

I can't tell you how many messages and emails I get from readers who say they'd love to do what I do with my fridge but their fridge is too small, too old, too gross, too dysfunctional, too you-name-it for them to make the effort. They say *when* they get a new fridge, *then* they're going to get organized.

I'm calling that out right here, right now.

If your fridge is keeping your food cold, then your fridge is perfect just the way it is. It is doing precisely what it was made to do.

You don't need to plop down $2,600 to have a beautiful, well-functioning fridge. I don't want you to wait until things are perfect on the outside of your fridge to take action on the inside. I want you to unabashedly love the fridge you're with, dents, stains, funkiness and all—I promise you we're going to make this work! I'm going to give you all the tools and techniques you need to turn the fridge you're lucky enough to own right now into the best possible fridge it can be. I'd much rather you invest in what goes *inside* your fridge than making sure it doesn't look dated on the outside.

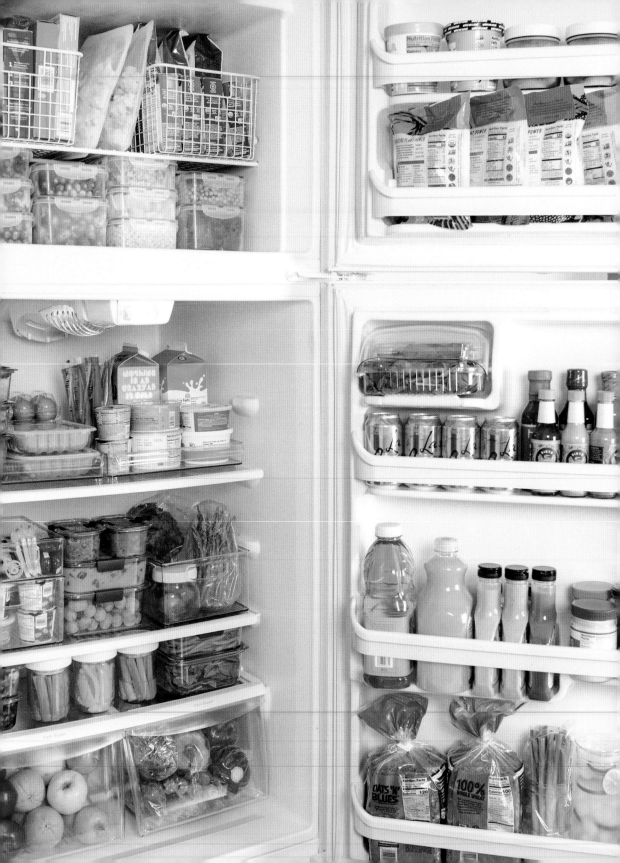

Let's say a big, fat, collective NO to conspicuous fridge consumption. It's not good for your wallet, and it's not good for the environment, either. Because there's one more bit of history I left till now to discuss.

There's a cost to our cold.

With every new technology comes a dark side—an unintended consequence of making life easier. For refrigeration, the drawback has been chemical refrigerants. The earliest refrigerants caused damage on the human level with explosions and poisoning. Then in the 1930s, a new refrigerant—chlorofluorocarbons (also known as CFCs, or the trademarked name Freon)—was put into widespread use and became the dominant refrigerant until the 1970s. But by the 1980s, scientists had identified these CFCs as contributing to the hole in the ozone layer. Refrigerants were being released when old refrigerators were crushed and buried, allowing the CFCs to escape into the atmosphere. In 1987, the world agreed to stop the use of CFCs in an international treaty called the Montreal Protocol.

So what refrigerant do fridge manufacturers use today? Perfluorocarbons (PFCs), which thankfully don't damage the ozone layer. That doesn't mean they aren't dangerous to the environment, however. In fact, PFCs are more potent greenhouse gases than carbon dioxide—trapping thousands of times more heat energy in the atmosphere. The good news is that when you properly dispose of your fridge (see below), refrigerants can safely be disposed of.

What Happens When Your Fridge Dies

Probably the most ecofriendly thing you can do when it comes to your fridge is to keep the fridge you have until it completely stops working. You'll get far more mileage from any fridge if you practice the airflow recommendations we covered later in the book.

When it's finally time to get rid of it, city and state regulations for disposal and/or recycling will vary; you'll need to check with your local agencies for guidelines. If you're buying a new fridge, the retailer may offer the option of hauling away your old one. Some charities may also accept donations of refrigerators in good working condition.

SELECTING YOUR FRIDGE GOAL(S)

We all want different things out of life, and it's the same when it comes to our fridges. The functions I expect my fridge to perform for my life and eating preferences are going to be different from yours. Identifying your goals will set realistic expectations of how your fridge will look and function.

A lot of readers say they want a fridge like mine, where they open the doors and immediately see a rainbow of fresh fruits and veggies. But when I press further, they tell me they don't want to dedicate hours to prep or that they eat a more processed diet. That means their goal is not realistic for their current time commitment and priorities. If you pursue a goal that doesn't align with your life as it is today or to which you're not going to dedicate the effort needed to change, it's going to leave you feeling frustrated and falling short.

I want to take some time now to help you determine how much advanced prep (if any) you'll want to do at the start of each week. We're going to base it on approximate time needed (remember, you'll get faster with practice), dietary preferences (more processed foods or more whole foods), and whether you prefer to cook each day or cook once for the week ahead. In other words, how do you want your fridge to serve you?

I've created four preparation-level-based goals and one values-based goal, established from the types of readers I've helped in my work with my blog, *Hello Nutritarian*. You should be able to find at least one goal that you identify with.

1. **The Fresh Fridge:** You're looking to organize your fridge and learn techniques to maximize produce freshness. The idea of opening your fridge and easily identifying ingredients inspires you. You're not particularly concerned about eliminating all processed foods, but you'd like to eat more fresh produce in general. You prefer on-demand cooking to meal prep. *Estimated time commitment:* 15 to 30 minutes per week

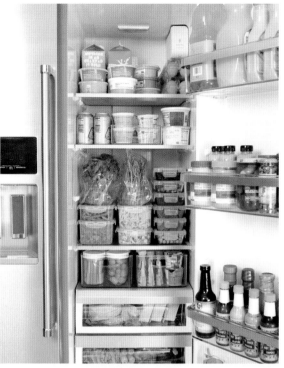

THE FRESH FRIDGE

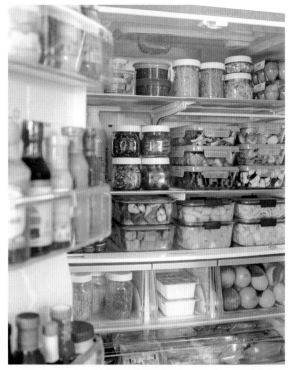

THE CHOPPED FRIDGE

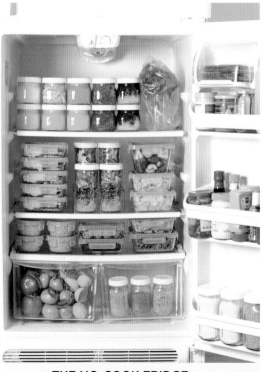

THE NO-COOK FRIDGE

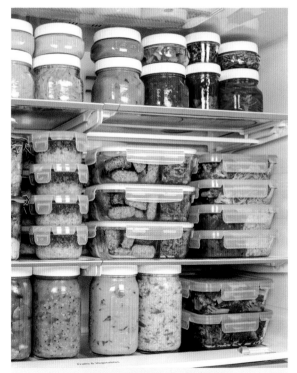

THE PREPPED FRIDGE

2. **The Chopped Fridge:** Fridge organization is a must, but you're really here to get your chop on! The idea of opening your fridge and finding cut fruits and veggies ready for healthy snacking, as well as chopped components so you can cook faster during the week appeals to you. You're a predominantly on-demand cooker. *Estimated time commitment:* 1 to 1½ hours per week

3. **The No-Cook Fridge:** You're not exactly ready to commit to batch cooking for the week, but you'd love to layer more easy-to-make no-cook preps into your Chopped Fridge practice. You can take an extra hour each week to make homemade sauces, components, and no-cook meals that can supplement the rest of your cooking during the week. *Estimated time commitment:* 1½ to 2 hours per week

4. **The Prepped Fridge:** You want to chop and cook all the things! You're willing to spend a few hours on the weekend to ensure a week of grab-and-go meals and healthy eating. Maybe you're taking on a new healthy lifestyle and need to put extra effort in up front to get it off the ground. You're very interested in prepping, but you may have little practical experience. In short, you've got great fridge-spectations! *Estimated time commitment:* 2 to 3 hours per week

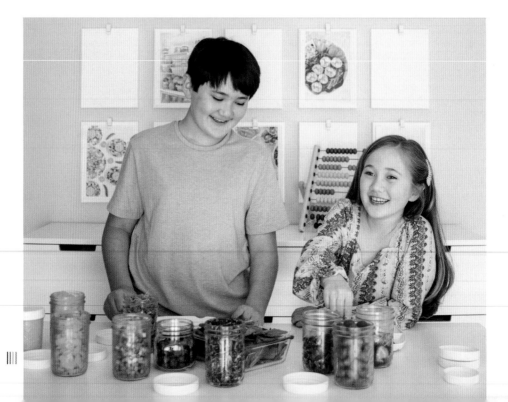

The Ecofriendly Fridge

You're viewing your lifestyle, eating, and storage solutions through the lens of minimizing your carbon footprint. You pay special attention to reducing plastic use and extending the mechanical life of your fridge. You're willing to spend extra time and energy to minimize food waste and make components from scratch to avoid excessive packaging and processed foods.

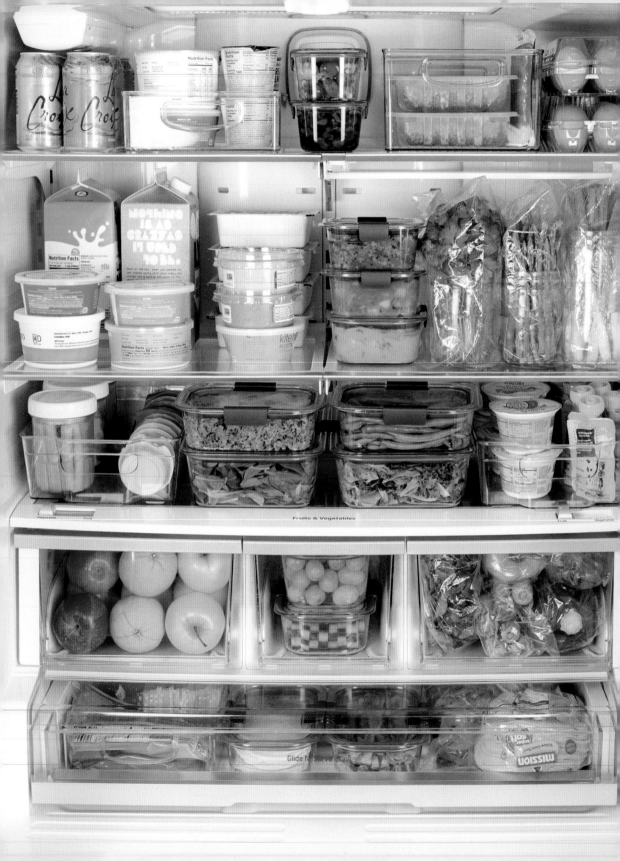

Part 2

FRIDGE SETTINGS, CLEANING, STORAGE, AND ORGANIZATION

I'm not expecting you to track down your fridge manual and read up on every single setting—I fully understand that not everyone is a raging fridge-geek like me. But I do want you to grasp the basics so you don't inadvertently get in the way of a good thing.

HOW YOUR FRIDGE WORKS

Refrigeration actually works by taking heat away from the inside of a compartment. The mechanisms in your fridge continuously pass a cold liquid around the objects to be cooled. Instead of "creating" artificial cold, the refrigeration system is continuously extracting heat. That's why you'll notice hot air coming out from the vents at the bottom or back of your fridge.

Your fridge is essentially moving heat around, using a gas refrigerant that expands and contracts to manipulate the temperature. The goal is to get heat into and back out of the refrigerant over and over again in a closed system.

The machinery that makes this refrigeration cycle happen has four major components:

1. **COMPRESSOR: INCREASES PRESSURE**
2. **CONDENSER: DISCHARGES HEAT**
3. **METERING DEVICE (USUALLY A CAPILLARY TUBE): DROPS PRESSURE**
4. **EVAPORATOR FAN: ABSORBS HEAT**

The refrigeration cycle is essentially absorbing heat, pressurizing the refrigerant, removing the heat, then dropping the pressure. Then the cycle repeats itself, continuously—your fridge is always in one of these phases of the cycle. The noises you hear from your fridge occur when one phase is triggered or ends.

The compressor can turn off when the refrigerator is at the correct temperature. But if the temperature starts to rise slightly, the compressor will kick back on and pump the refrigerant through the cycle again.

If the compressor is running, the condenser fan is also running, pumping refrigerant through the condenser coils. The condenser fan is responsible for cooling the refrigerant as it flows through the condenser coils, dispelling the heat picked up inside the box, and returning the refrigerant to a liquid.

The evaporator fan's motor is always running, even if the compressor and condenser fan are off. The evaporator fan is responsible for keeping a constant flow of air in the refrigerator box. It must keep the air moving and flowing over the evaporator coils so the refrigerant can absorb the heat from inside the fridge.

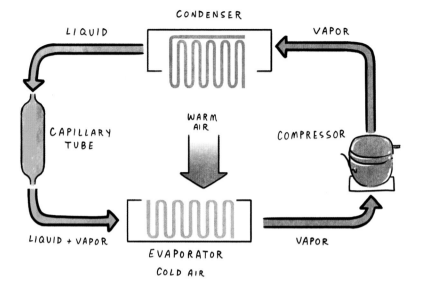

CONDENSER
LIQUID   VAPOR
CAPILLARY
TUBE
WARM
AIR
COMPRESSOR
LIQUID + VAPOR   VAPOR
EVAPORATOR
COLD AIR

Since frost accumulates on the supercooled condenser coils, an automatic defrost heater is a standard feature on modern fridges. This heater is usually a simple wire filament enclosed within a tube that has electricity running through the wire. It heats the tube and melts the frost on the coils, sending the melted water to a drip pan that catches the liquid and condensation, which eventually evaporates from the pan.

Now, if there's only one thing you take away from any of this, let it be this: heat triggers the refrigeration cycle to begin. If heat is making its way into your fridge, your energy use goes up and the environment in your fridge changes. And heat makes its way in every time you open the doors or add warm food to the fridge.

Temperature Is Everything

Keeping your food at optimal storage temperatures is the number one factor in lengthening its shelf life. That's why a fridge's job is to keep heat out.

Your goal is to make sure your fridge can do its best work. Fostering optimal conditions in your fridge ensures that it can maintain a constant temperature.

You do this by understanding these three aspects of refrigerated temperature:

- How airflow works and locating the critical airflow areas of your particular fridge
- Best practices for adjusting temperature settings
- How humidity impacts maintaining that ideal temperature
  Now we're really digging into the good stuff . . .

Understanding Airflow

Your refrigerator relies on forced air to transfer heat. Internal fans move air around the inside of your fridge. The faster that air flows, the more quickly heat is removed. For this reason, you don't want to do anything to block the airflow.

Each fridge has a different airflow arrangement based on its price and included features. I'm going to provide specific configuration (side-by-side, freezer-top, etc.) information for you starting on page 22, but for now let's just cover the basic principles of fridge airflow.

There are three basic types of airflow systems in refrigerators:

1. **Ceiling-type airflow:** A single fan is mounted on the ceiling of the appliance. Found in older or basic fridge models.
2. **Back wall– or mullion-type airflow:** The airflow system takes in air above the top shelf and discharges it below the bottom shelf. Found in many midrange models.
3. **Duct-type airflow:** A combination of the first two types, where the forced-air unit is located at or above ceiling level, and the air is circulated through a series of small air ducts vented to various spots on the back wall of the cabinet. Found in newer, higher-end models.

Typically, your refrigerator section gets its cold air from the freezer section. The air flows in a circular pattern between the refrigerator and the freezer. If you were to take the backplate off your freezer section, you'd see the evaporator is a frosted-up coil (which houses that magical refrigerant) with a fan that sucks air across the coils and into the freezer compartment.

Depending on your model, your fridge might have sensors, a timer, a general thermostat, or a combination of these components, which signal how much of the cold freezer air should be diverted into the refrigerated compartment. This is typically regulated by a damper—a vent, flap, or fan between the refrigerator and freezer sections.

The damper is the heart of airflow in your fridge—it pumps and circulates cooled air throughout. Different fridge models handle airflow differently (ceiling-, back wall-, or duct-type) but here's a general breakdown.

In basic fridge models, the damper vent is the only point of entry for cool air into the refrigerated compartment, so it's responsible for all the cooling and circulation that happens within. It's a really good idea, especially if you have an older or more basic model fridge, to find where the damper vent is in your particular unit. If you don't have your fridge manual anymore, the damper is usually found in the top of the fridge or on the back panel near the top.

Cold air moves from the damper down the back of your fridge. That's why the coldest parts of your fridge are the top shelf and toward the back of your shelves (we'll put this knowledge to use when we talk about organization). As the cooled air travels down your fridge, it's diverted to each shelf. Then it's sucked in by another hole near the bottom of the refrigerator section. That air is then drawn in by some vents at the bottom of the evaporator. It's sucked back over the frosted-up coils of the evaporator, cooling the air again, and the cycle starts over.

Typically, the coldest parts of your fridge include:

- the top shelf, near the damper vent
- the back wall of your fridge
- near airflow vents
- the back area of each shelf

Typically, the warmer parts of your fridge include:

- door storage
- the front of your shelves nearest the doors
- crisper drawers

IDENTIFYING *YOUR* CRITICAL AIRFLOW POINTS

Now I want you to get hands-on for a sec. Get on up and head over to your fridge, and let's figure out the kind of airflow you're working with. This is extra important if you've ever had any concerns about the cooling capacity of your fridge.

Locate the damper vent (as described on page 21) and test the airflow by holding your hand up to it for a few seconds. If you don't feel anything, don't freak out! Certain models will close the damper when the fridge door is open. Just hold down the light switch or tape it so the fridge thinks the door is closed.

Next, follow the path of the air and see which areas of your fridge get the most airflow and which get the least. Notice how the air is forced to go into ever-smaller spaces as it heads to the drawers. Finally, locate where the air is being sucked back in, toward the bottom of the unit.

As I've said before, our job is to not get in the way of a good thing. Actually feeling your fridge's airflow will help keep you mindful of minimizing block-ages along that path (especially important if you're working with an older or basic model fridge).

Basic Freezer-Top Fridges

The damper, or hole from the freezer, is housed at the top back of the fridge. It pushes the cooled air along the back wall of the fridge compartment.

If you notice the back of your shelves have a raised finlike indentation, this subtle aerodynamic design addition allows the main column of air to get diverted off onto each shelf area. It's really critical with a fridge design like this to keep at least 4 inches of clear space from the back lip of the shelf to ensure airflow is coming across your shelf and making its way toward the front of the unit.

Depending on your model, you may notice a series of vents at the very back of your crisper drawers. They are shaped in a way that helps divert some airflow to the bottom shelf and the remaining airflow to the sides of the crisper drawers (along the side walls of the fridge). You'll find manual sliders that say "LO" and "HI" that allow more or less air into the drawers. The crisper drawers are the most humid parts of your fridge because they restrict airflow so much.

Side-by-Side Fridges

The damper vent is usually housed at the top left corner section of your fridge compartment. Some models will have a flap and others will have a covered mechanized damper fan spanning the hole in the wall between the freezer and fridge sections.

Airflow in basic side-by-side models will be the same as basic freezer-top units (described above), it's just the location of the airflow source that's different. But more expensive side-by-side models will offer airflow improvements using back wall- or duct-type configurations. Some of these pricier models will have airflow vents at every shelf interval. Others will have a raised column on the back wall of the fridge that has vents pointing airflow out and curving around the fridge compartment walls.

Again, it's important to identify your particular airflow source so you can make sure to keep those areas of your fridge clear.

French Door Models

Typically, French door–model fridges contain higher-end features by default. When it comes to airflow, this usually means a duct-type configuration with more sensors in more areas of the fridge, allowing for more targeted airflow release. This also means more airflow spigots arranged over more parts of the fridge—if airflow is impeded in one area, that area can effectively be bypassed so air will continue to be released in another area.

These bells and whistles aren't necessary for an optimally running fridge; they just make it harder for you to screw things up if you know zero about fridge airflow. But that's definitely not you anymore!

DUAL-EVAPORATOR MODELS

Starting around 2013, one of the biggest innovations in fridge airflow has been the mechanical upgrade to two (or lately even three) evaporators. A quick refresher: The evaporator is that frosted coil that's pulling heat out of the unit and providing the source of cool air. The latest fridge models have separate cooling sources (evaporators) for both the freezer compartment and the fridge compartment.

Having two different evaporators can be quite helpful if you want to opti-mize the heck out of your fridge. Dual-evaporative refrigerators create two distinct climates: colder, dryer air in the freezer and warmer, more humid air in the fridge.

This feature spans all configurations (freezer-top, side-by-side, and French door) but isn't standard on all fridges. If you happen to have a dual-evaporator model—they really started to get popular around 2016—then you have another layer of optimization when it comes to airflow. This feature has also allowed some manufacturers to add specialized fridge modes like "vacation" or "half full." And many of the latest models even let you convert the freezer section to fresh storage as needed!

Temperature Settings

Choosing the target temperature for your fridge is setting a goal for your machine. The temperature you set tells the compressor when to turn on or start a new cycle. When the temperature rises above that number, the system knows there's heat that needs to be extracted.

Deciding what temperature to set your fridge to can be tricky. The USDA has determined 37°F to be most protective against food spoilage and food-borne illnesses. As a general rule of thumb, a fridge over 40°F (or a freezer over 5°F) is too warm, and most fridge units won't go below 33°F, so you have a range of about 7 degrees to play with.

Higher-end fridges have lots of sensors that constantly send feedback to the system so it can adjust the overall temperature for different zones in the fridge. But basic models have only a knob that you can set somewhere between "cold" and "coldest," so you may not know when 37°F is actually being reached. While every fridge model comes with recommended tempera-ture settings (even the knob-only fridges have "factory setting" or "recom-mended" positions), this may not be sufficient given the climate and ambient conditions where you live. If you have an older fridge or basic model, I recom-mend using a thermometer to monitor the temperature of the unit. You can get a reliable refrigerator thermometer for about $10.

Airflow goes hand in hand with the accuracy and effectiveness of your temperature setting. Blocked air vents can cause temperature inconsistencies, fluctuations, and unintentional freezing. Always remember that you're going to get the most accurate temperature from a fridge that has optimized air circulation.

It's also important to note that the temperature in your unit will fluctuate. This typically happens as the refrigerator goes through a defrost cycle (when a small heater dissolves the frost buildup around the evaporator coils). If you notice that the internal temperature seems high, wait an hour or so to see if it moderates.

Don't be afraid to adjust your temperature settings. For example, I change the temp in my fridge—a 2013 LG French door model—throughout the week to account for my weekly meal prepping. After I've prepped my foods for the week and stored them in the fridge, I set the temperature to 38°F, because that's what I've found to work best. If I'm looking to extend my prepped foods for longer than a week, I'll lower the temp to 37°F. I keep my freezer at 3°F. Because the airflow in my fridge is strong and certain areas around the air vents are prone to freezing, my preferred temps may be a little higher than yours. If you have a temperature that works for you, keep it as is and focus instead on maximizing your airflow.

If you do change the temperature, wait at least 24 hours before lowering it another degree or setting. This allows your fridge to run enough cycles for the new temperature setting to take effect. Be warned that drastic temperature changes can lead to freezing—you don't want to accidentally freeze your latest grocery haul.

Humidity

When it comes to the microclimate in your fridge, it's important to understand the interaction between temperature and humidity.

Humidity is the moisture content in the air, and the humidity levels in your fridge are always proportionate to the unit's interior temperature. Lowering the temperature decreases air's ability to hold moisture—so air is made drier by cooling it. That's why we spent time learning about airflow and gauging the right temperature for your unit—those are going to be your first lines of defense against the onslaught of excess humidity.

Depending on the climate where you live, battling humidity in your fridge may be an everyday reality. A person in a humid climate can have a drastically different fridge experience than someone living in a dry environment. The good news is, there are ways to maintain optimal humidity.

Two important aspects of humidity are how your fridge regulates moisture and sources of moisture inside your fridge. Understanding these factors will help you make the best of your particular fridge-climate dynamic.

FRIDGE-GENERATED HUMIDITY

Air can hold different amounts of water at different temperatures. When it comes to refrigeration, the type of humidity we are interested in is relative humidity, or what percentage of its maximum water-holding capacity the air contains at any given time. For example, 75 percent relative humidity means the air is holding 75 percent as much water as it could at that temperature.

Remember, in most fridge models, cool air is diverted from the freezer compartment to the fridge compartment. When the air is drawn over the cooling coils, which are below freezing, any moisture is drawn out and condensed into ice crystals. Freezers maintain an average relative humidity of only 30 to 35 percent. The low relative humidity is important in the freezer section because any more moisture in the air would cause excessive frost on the evaporator coils, leading to airflow blockages.

Refrigerators create cool, dry air. But dry air isn't a good thing for your refrigerated foods, and especially not for produce. Most foods do best at 80 to 85 percent relative humidity. Fresh produce is even more water-needy: Up to 95 percent relative humidity is ideal to keep produce fresh and crisp.

Your fridge can't introduce any moisture into its environment on its own. So how do you take the cold, dry air from the freezer and make it optimal for foods stored in the fridge? The only way to increase the moisture content in the refrigerator compartment is to slow down air circulation. That's why crisper drawers were one of the earliest features added to home fridge units.

These closed produce bins help hold in natural moisture from your produce and restrict the flow of dry, cool air.

As you can see, refrigeration is a delicate balancing act between airflow, temperature, and humidity.

You can buy a humidity sensor for your fridge, but here are a few signs to help you gauge if its relative humidity is higher than the optimal 80 to 85 percent range:

- Moisture buildup on the walls and/or shelves in the fridge compartment
- Moisture buildup concentrated in a particular location in the fridge compartment
- Frost or ice buildup along the walls and/or shelves in the freezer compartment

EXTERNALLY INTRODUCED SOURCES OF HUMIDITY

If your fridge is dank, wet, and full of condensation, the answer is not that you need a new fridge! If the mechanical components of the fridge are in good working order, and air is circulating efficiently without blockages, your sad, wet state of affairs is likely because of what's getting *into* your fridge, not the fridge itself.

Internal fridge humidity is influenced by these factors, in order of importance:

- How often you open your fridge doors
- The climate you live in, especially the environment in the immediate area around your fridge (also known as the ambient conditions)
- An ineffective door seal
- Airflow blockages
- Putting warm or hot food in the unit
- Putting too much room-temperature food in at one time
- Putting too many wet foods in the unit
- Storing too many open containers (especially beverages)

The number one factor in keeping a consistent temperature and humidity level in your fridge is how frequently you open the doors. How much moisture gets in when you open the doors is directly linked to the climate you live in, the time of year, and the humidity in the air immediately surrounding your fridge.

For example, a few years ago we took a family vacation to Hawaii—and stayed in a vacation rental without air-conditioning. The main reason we rented a house was so we could eat in as much as possible. I couldn't understand why the same foods I would prep for myself at home weren't lasting as long in Hawaii. It wasn't until I compiled my research for this book that I finally understood: Whenever I opened the fridge in our Hawaiian "hothouse" during the afternoon, I was pretty much blasting the inside of the fridge with air that had 100 percent relative humidity. This taxed the fridge system, forcing it to work harder to do its job. The result was that the freezer felt like the refrigerated compartment should have, and the refrigerated compartment felt like a wet, slightly melted ice pop. Had I known what I know today, I would have been vigilant about minimizing door openings, especially during the hottest times of day. At least until the unit had enough time to figuratively catch its breath.

Here's all the best advice I've collected on how to minimize humidity in your fridge.

- Organize your fridge so you can quickly pick out the foods you need and minimize how long the doors stay open (don't worry—there's lots of organization goodness to come). Limit how frequently you open the doors during excessively hot or humid weather or times of day.

- Remember, your fridge is extracting heat from its interior, and that displaced heat is then released into the surrounding area. Make sure your refrigerator isn't pushed right up against a wall; leave at least 4 inches between the wall and the back of the refrigerator so air can circulate freely and better disperse heat from the condenser. If you can, situate your fridge in a cool place with plenty of space around it so that heat can dissipate faster. If rearranging the room isn't an option, adding a fan or two to your kitchen area can help lower the ambient humidity.

- Check to ensure that the gasket—the soft rubber or plastic seal that surrounds your fridge doors—has a tight fit. You can do this by holding a small piece of paper against the doorframe and closing the door. If you can pull the paper out easily, the gasket may need replacing.

- Keep the grill of your unit free of dust and lint to permit air to flow freely to the condenser. The grill may be housed in the front or back of your fridge, depending on the model.

- Make sure to identify the airflow areas of your fridge (as outlined on page 22) and keep those areas clear of large items.

- Most fridge manufacturers recommend that you let cooked food cool completely before putting it in the fridge. Never put uncovered warm food directly into the fridge, as the warm air will create condensation.

- Adding too many room-temperature items to your fridge at once makes your refrigerator have to work harder to extract heat and cool the space. For example, avoid stuffing your fridge with twenty-five room-temperature bottles of water or soda cans at once. If you're battling too much interior moisture, add only enough items as you'll need for the next day or two.

- Your groceries can introduce moisture, so make sure to wipe any external water from bags or packages before placing them in the fridge or freezer, and dry off wet produce before storing it, or place paper towels in the crisper drawers to absorb excess moisture.

- Open containers of food or beverages let moisture into your fridge compartment. If you don't plan on consuming the food or drink within three to four hours, make sure to cover those items.

- Use a food-grade desiccant dehumidifier in your refrigerator. These use a material, most commonly silica gel, that extracts and holds water vapor. These come in small boxes, canisters, or bags and are typically used in closets, safes, and bathrooms but will work in a refrigerator, too.

- Create more space between your food. Keep containers at least 1 inch away from each other to encourage airflow.

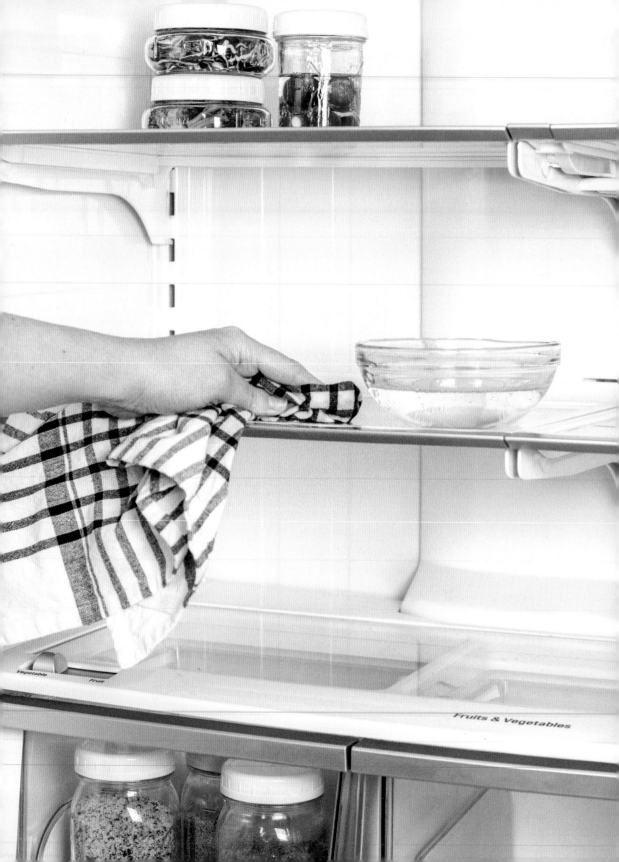

CLEANING YOUR FRIDGE

Did you know that depending on where you live, it can cost over $300 to have your fridge cleaned? Just think of that the next time you take on the task! If this sounds like just about the last thing you want to do, why not incentivize yourself with splurging on some new food storage containers as a reward for going that extra mile and getting your fridge looking its Sunday best?

Cleaning the fridge is an instant mood-lifter (after all, you have to look at it every single day) and stress-buster (nothing makes me feel more in control than sparkling-clean shelves). Not to mention, it keeps you and your family safe from unwanted microorganisms like bacteria, mold, and yeast that can ruin your food and potentially compromise your health. And honestly, there's no more manageable makeover you can do as a weekend house project! Read on to learn what to do and when to do it.

THE DEEP CLEAN

What is it? Taking everything out of your fridge and cleaning every surface.

- **How long will it take?** Depending on when you performed your last cleaning, how large your fridge is, and how many components your particular fridge model has, this can take anywhere from 1 to 2 hours.

- **When should I do it?** I provide two sample deep-cleaning schedules on page 35, but because a deep clean means taking all the food out of your fridge, as a general rule I always recommend doing it right before you go grocery shopping, when you have the lowest stock of food. Another ideal time to deep clean is right before you go on a vacation—it's a great way to get rid of perishable items and come home to a clean slate.

How to do it:

- **If this is your very first deep clean:** Start with a little planning before you actually get cleaning. You want to have read through the organization section (starting on page 36) and decided which food storage containers you'll use going forward. Choose a goal (see page 12) so you'll have a clear idea what you'll be picking up on your next grocery run and how you'll restock your fridge after this deep clean.

- **Where do I put the food while I clean?** I like to hold the food in a cooler. You can add ice if you have perishable foods; if it's mostly condiments and beverages, they will be fine in the insulated cooler while you work. Just make sure to wipe down and dry everything you put back into your cleaned fridge.

- **Do I turn off my fridge?** If you haven't done a deep clean in over a year, I would recommend turning off your fridge while you work. There have likely been internal spills that may require some extra time and elbow grease to remove. I recommend waiting until after you've finished removing and washing the fridge components (see below) before unplugging the fridge. If you've done a deep clean within the last year and/or you don't see any major areas of concern, it's fine to leave the unit on while you clean. Just make sure to shut the doors after you remove the components to wash them (see below). If you've turned off your fridge, be sure to keep the freezer shut, without opening it at all, while you're working in order to retain as much cold as possible. (If you want to clean your freezer, do it on a different day to avoid overtaxing your refrigerator, and keep the unit *on*.)

- **Start by removing the fridge shelves, drawers, and door storage components and washing them:** Pretty much, if it isn't nailed down, you want to remove it and clean it! This is the most critical component of a deep clean because that's where you'll find spills that have gone unnoticed and any microbial growth that may have resulted. This is also a great time to check the mechanical components of your fridge and identify your model's airflow (as described on page 22). If this is your first time removing these pieces, you might want to snap a quick picture beforehand to remind you where everything goes. Remove all the components at once—this will minimize opening and closing of the fridge doors. Wash each piece in the sink with warm water and soap. If you're battling any smells in your fridge, adding a bit of baking soda when washing is helpful. Lay the components out on a large towel to dry while you clean the interior of the fridge, then use a dish towel to dry any remaining moisture on the clean components—this will give your fridge compartment time to dry and cool down again if the unit has been on. Make sure everything is completely dry before putting the components back in the fridge.

- **Cleaning the interior:** Use a clean rag dipped in a mixture of water and dish soap; an easy recipe is 3 cups warm water mixed with 2 teaspoons dish soap. You can also add up to 2 tablespoons baking soda to help eliminate odors. If you're encountering particularly stubborn, sticky spills, feel free to use a chemical cleaning spray to help lift off the residue—just try not to spray down the whole interior, as the chemicals can linger and settle on food. Start by cleaning the ceiling of the refrigerator compartment, then work your way down the sides. Pay close attention to bracket holders and corners, where crumbs and debris can accumulate. Clean around the drawer frames and finish by wiping down the interior of the fridge doors. Use a few dry dish towels to dry the interior after cleaning, then return the clean, dry components to their positions.

- **Editing your food:** Now that the fridge is all clean and dry, it's time to put your food back inside. This is the perfect time to edit out foods that are expired or no longer serve your health goals. Condiments are a critical category, as they are most likely to be expired. If you bought a special condiment for a certain recipe but haven't used it since, it's time to say goodbye. In fact, if you haven't used something in the past 6 months, it's time to let it go to make room for foods you want to eat daily.

- **Rest period:** Now that everything is clean and you've edited your food, it's a good idea to let the fridge rest for at least an hour before you put any *new* food in there. (It's perfectly fine to return the food that you kept in the cooler to the fridge; this food should still be cool.) If you had to turn off your unit, you'll want to just let it be for about 3 hours before you add new food or open the doors—remember, the unit will be working harder to process the heat that entered during cleaning.

WEEKLY WIPE DOWNS

What is it? A weekly check-in to spot clean any areas of concern, discard old items, and monitor conditions to know when you'll need to do your next deep clean.

- **How long will this take?** No more than 20 minutes.

- **When do I do it?** Again, the best time for any kind of fridge cleaning is right before you go grocery shopping, when your fridge is the most empty.

How to do it:

- **Do I turn off my fridge?** No, you'll only be wiping down the shelves and inside the drawers.

- **Where do I put the food?** There's no need to remove everything. I like to start at the top, moving everything down to the shelf below and wiping down the top shelf. Then I put food back on the shelf and continue down the compartment in that fashion.

- **What do I clean with?** You can use a slightly dampened clean rag or sponge.

- **Where do I clean?** Focus on cleaning just the shelves and drawers. Nothing needs to be removed at this time.

MAINTENANCE CLEANING SCHEDULE

Let's answer a question I get asked a whole lot: How often should you deep clean the fridge? Keeping your fridge clean is a mixture of weekly wipe downs and more intensive deep cleans. The right balance depends on the size of your family and frequency of use.

Q1: END OF THE FIRST WEEK OF JANUARY

Q2: END OF THE FIRST WEEK OF APRIL

Q3: END OF THE FIRST WEEK OF JULY*

Q4: END OF THE FIRST WEEK OF OCTOBER

*Q3 Note: If you live in an area with particularly hot and humid summers or have issues with moisture in your fridge during this time of year, feel free to skip this deep cleaning. It's more important to keep the temperature of your unit stable than to clean it to this degree. Just be sure to keep up your deep cleaning during the rest of the year.

This option is best for families of four or more with lots of daily fridge usage. Because there are more people reaching into the fridge, there are more opportunities for spills and accumulation of dust, crumbs, and hair. If you fall into this category, I recommend deep cleaning your fridge quarterly. This is the cleaning schedule I personally follow, and I love the seasonality of it—just before and after the holidays are prime fridge-cleaning times because of the added holiday cooking and family gatherings.

Supplement your quarterly deep cleans with weekly wipe downs. You pretty much want to wipe things down before you bring new food in. If you go longer than a week between food shopping, feel free to space out your wipe downs accordingly.

BIANNUAL SCHEDULE

DEEP CLEANING 1: END OF THE FIRST WEEK OF APRIL

DEEP CLEANING 2: END OF THE FIRST WEEK OF OCTOBER

This option is best for households with three or fewer people and/or very light fridge usage. Supplement with weekly wipe downs as you would with the quarterly schedule above.

FRIDGE ORGANIZATION

I see fridge organization as the perfect marriage of function and motivation. Good organization helps you find things easily, so you're not wasting time with your fridge doors open (which wastes money in the form of energy use, ages your unit, and shortens the shelf life of your food). And the aesthetics of a beautifully organized refrigerator motivate us to want to eat in and eat fresh, as we're drawn to the attractively showcased ingredients. Like a gorgeously decorated dessert, a well-dressed fridge invites us to take a bite!

MY THREE GUIDING PRINCIPLES TO FRIDGE ORGANIZATION
No matter which goal(s) you identified for yourself on page 12, these guiding organization principles will help you most in getting there.

1. FRONT OF FRIDGE, FRONT OF MIND.
2. THINK OUTSIDE THE CRISPER DRAWERS.
3. LESS IS ACTUALLY MORE.

Front of Fridge, Front of Mind
This is my number one most important organization principle. We eat with our eyes, so you want to make sure the foods you actually *want* to eat are the first thing you see when you open your fridge. If you have a goal to eat more dark leafy greens, then that's what you should be seeing the most of when you open your fridge. If your goal is to get more produce into your diet, you want to make it as accessible as possible. Showcase the most nutritious foods your fridge has to offer, and make it as convenient as possible to eat them.

Depending on your goal(s), this could look like peeling and chopping some carrots, arranging them in a glass jar, and setting them on an eye-level shelf. How much more likely are you to reach for those carrots in the next three days than if they were languishing in your crisper drawer in the bag in which you brought them home from the grocery store? And even if you're more the chop-as-you-go type, taking the time to arrange the whole carrots (skin-on, with the greens attached) upright in a container at the front of your

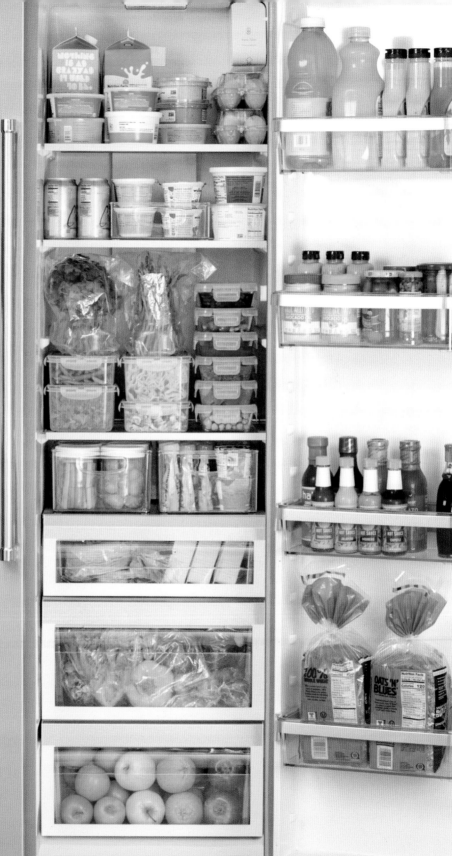
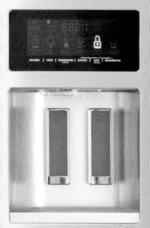

fridge where you'll see them immediately is, again, a great way to showcase that ingredient.

The goals are to take down the barriers to use and create opportunities for instant meal inspiration. You put your "best food forward" when you:

- Pull forward the foods that you want to be eating more of each day.
- Make those foods immediately visible to you when you open the fridge (stored in clear containers at eye level).
- Remember that your intention is to inspire your future self to want to eat or cook with those foods.

Think Outside the Crisper Drawers

The contents of your fridge should reflect your food pyramid. If you're looking to eat 50 percent unprocessed fruits and vegetables, then 50 percent of your fridge space should be dedicated to those foods. The crisper drawers account for only about 20 percent of the available real estate in a fridge (and that's a liberal estimate)—and 20 percent just isn't enough.

I aim to eat at least 75 percent unprocessed fruits and veggies. (The other 25 percent of my diet includes herbs, beans, whole grains, raw nuts and seeds, and tofu or tempeh.) It would be impossible for me to fit all the produce I need for the week in the limited space provided by my crisper drawer.

The good news is that you can re-create the humid conditions of your crisper drawers with the right food storage containers (we'll be getting to that soon). The point here is to not confine yourself to the given zones in your fridge. By understanding the airflow functions of your particular model, coupled with tightly sealed food storage containers, you'll see that you can treat *so* much more of your fridge like your crisper drawers!

Less Is More

I'm sure you've heard that the cure for "I don't have anything to wear" is actually to edit down your wardrobe to the pieces you wear and love the most. The magic of the capsule closet is that the fewer clothes you have to choose from, the easier it is to put together outfits. Well, the same is true of the food you put in your fridge.

Americans tend to fall into the overbuying-food trap because we happen to have the largest fridges in the world—as of 2002, US fridges averaged 28.6 cubic feet in volume. As fridge historian Jonathan Rees puts it in his book *Refrigerator*, "While Americans don't really need all this space inside their refrigerators, the more space they have, the more likely it becomes that consumers in the United States will buy larger quantities of mass-produced food." The truth is, all this space compels us to "fill 'er up." But buying and storing more food in your fridge, especially in the form of large, boxed processed foods, keeps your fridge from being able to keep all your food the freshest it can be.

Remember, your fridge's temperature, the most critical factor in lengthening the shelf life of your food, is dependent on proper airflow. You'll have much stronger airflow, and thus better fridge performance, when you keep the amount of food in your fridge edited down—with ample room for air to flow behind, around, and over containers. Less food means fresher food.

So how do you put this into practice? Try not to go two rows back on any given shelf. I like to view my fridge in one dimension, with a single row of different foods on each shelf. I'll only add a second row if I have backstock of the same item. When I can open my fridge doors and see everything I have available to me at one glance, without having to move anything to see what's behind it, I can make fast decisions on what I'm going to eat or make.

Organize your fridge drawers in the same spirit. When you pull open a drawer, you want to easily see everything at once, either from the outside of the drawer (for shallower drawers) or from above (for deeper drawers). With a deep drawer, I like to use silicone bags for storage, so when I look down into the drawer, I can see all the foods at once, as if I'm looking into the drawer of a filing cabinet, and easily grab what I need.

I know this rule feels alarmingly counterintuitive. One of the biggest complaints I hear from readers is that there's not enough space in their fridges. But I believe that by aligning what you put into your fridge with your health goals (by stocking your fridge according to your food pyramid) and learning best practices for food storage, you'll see that less is most certainly more.

Understanding the Different Stages of Your Fridge

Just like you, the inside of your fridge changes daily. It is going to look drastically different throughout the week. There's a good reason I almost always post photos of my fridge after it's fully prepped—because that's when it's all dolled up!

I love taking pictures of my fridge in its Sunday best because I'm proud of myself for making the decision to practice fridge love as self-love again that week. My obligatory "shelfie" (as it's become known on the 'gram) is a victory lap. It's a visual celebration of putting myself and my eating goals first and knowing that the week ahead will be full of all the good things!

But the truth is, my fridge only looks that pristine for about 2 hours each week. So what does my fridge look like the day before grocery shopping and the day I go grocery shopping, and how is the food used up during the week?

Here's how I manage my fridge in flux, broken down into four stages:

Stage 1: BEFORE FOOD SHOPPING
Stage 2: AFTER FOOD SHOPPING
Stage 3: AFTER PROCESSING THE GROCERIES
Stage 4: MIDWEEK FLUX

Stage 1: Before Food Shopping

The goals during this stage, usually a day or two before you head back to the grocery store, are to take stock of what you need from the store and to prepare the fridge for this next influx of items. Cleaning and rearranging are key during this stage. Your fridge is at its emptiest point, so this is the time of week where you'll want to do a weekly wipe down or deep clean (as outlined on pages 31–35).

This is also the perfect time to check your airflow and temperature settings. During this stage, because there's less food in the fridge, I like to raise the temperature by 1°F, so the fridge isn't needlessly working quite so hard (I only recommend this for duct-type airflow configurations). Your food will stay adequately cooled because, by this point in the week, it's being housed a bit farther back on each shelf (see Stage 4: Midweek Flux, on page 44).

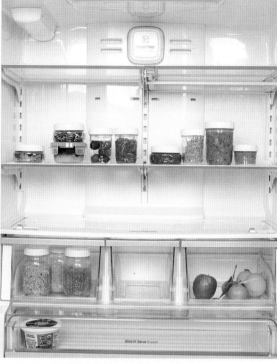

BEFORE FOOD SHOPPING

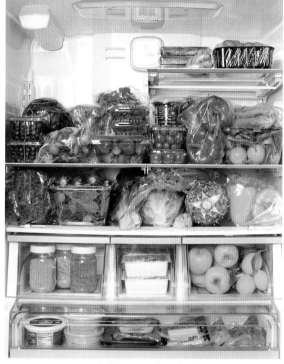

AFTER FOOD SHOPPING

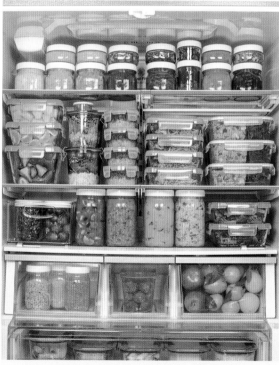

AFTER PROCESSING GROCERIES

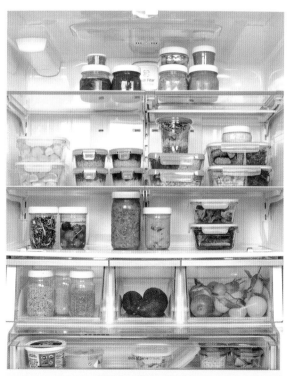

MIDWEEK FLUX

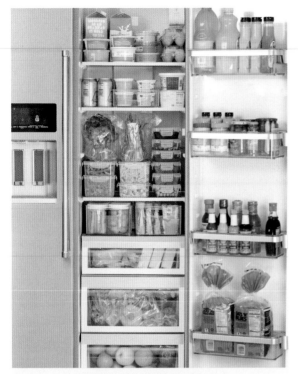

STORAGE PROCESSING

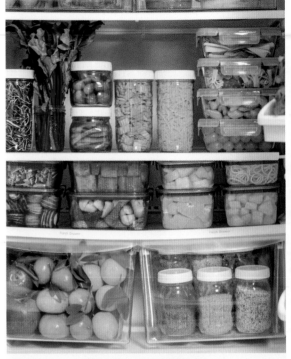

FRESH-PROCESSING

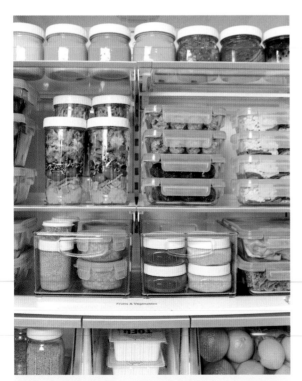

NO-COOK PREPS OR MIXING PROCESSING

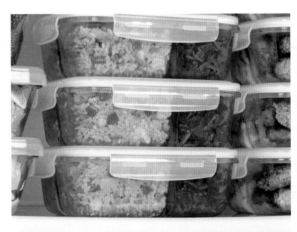

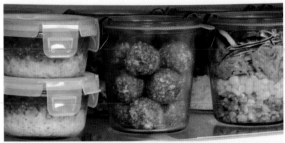

COOKED PREPS OR COOKING PROCESSING

Stage 2: After Food Shopping

This is when your fridge feels the most stuffed, because everything is in its whole state with its original packaging. You don't want your produce to go more than 24 hours in this state, since having things haphazardly piled up impedes airflow. I generally like to go food shopping one day, then "process" everything (meaning prep it for storage) over the next two days. This way the produce can cool off before it's washed and cut, reducing condensation in your storage containers and temperature fluctuations in your fridge.

By "processing" produce I mean reorganizing, prepping, and/or cooking it before storing it for use later in the week; which techniques you use will depend on your goals (see page 12) for any given week. (I share the best ways to store whole and prepped fruits and vegetables starting on page 88.) Your "After Processing" fridge (see Step 3) will look different based on the level of processing you do.

The Four Types/Levels of Processing

1. **Storage processing:** Storing whole produce in optimal conditions for maximum longevity and on-demand cooking inspiration. This usually means leaving it unwashed, with the skin on. This doesn't require much more than removing any damaged leaves, pieces, or parts and making sure everything is stored in ideal containers and locations in your fridge.

2. **Fresh-processing:** This means washing, peeling, trimming, and chopping fresh produce to make it more convenient to eat and/or cook during the week. Think of this as your *mise en place*, a culinary term for having all the components of a recipe chopped and easily accessible before you start cooking.

3. **No-cook preps or mixing processing:** This might involve making blended sauces and mixing together fresh ingredients for no-cooking-required preps throughout the week.

4. **Cooked preps or cooking processing:** Batch cooking some recipes for the week. You'll usually do this along with any no-cook preps and fresh-processing produce for the week.

Where you store your food after you're done processing is important. Keep things you want to eat or cook soon clearly visible, at eye level and in front.

If you're meal prepping, dishes you plan on eating later in the week should be stored closest to your airflow points, where the temperature is colder (typically toward the back; see page 22 if you need a refresher).

Stage 3: After Processing

This is when your fridge is in its most beautiful, vibrant state. Space has been cleared after grocery shopping because foods have been processed and put into containers. This is when you'll be doing the most organizing, following the guidelines beginning on page 36. This pristinely organized stage typically lasts 1 to 2 days, after which you'll find yourself in . . .

Stage 4: Midweek Flux

These are the 5 to 7 days where you're eating from your fridge before your next grocery shop. The most important thing to remember during this stage is first in, first out (FIFO)—or as I sometimes like to think of it, FSFO: first to spoil, first out.

You want to eat the food with the shortest shelf life (like fresh berries, cut bell peppers, and delicate greens) in the beginning of the week, and eat sturdier produce or long-keeping foods (red cabbage, carrots, some no-cook and/or cooked meal components) toward the end of the week.

As your fridge is in flux, you'll want to do some regular reorganization (you're going to have a lot more space to work with on day 4 than you did on day 1), using these two key strategies:

1. **Condensing down food containers:** This is one of the most valuable tips I can share for maximizing your food budget. You want as little air as possible between your food and the storage container, so use the smallest container that still fits the food. After you've eaten some of any particular food, transfer what's left into a smaller container (you don't want your containers to be less than 50 percent full for more than a day or two). This goes for cooked foods, chopped fresh produce, and sauces or homemade condiments. This is going to lengthen your food's shelf life and ensure freshness toward the end of the week. This will also create more space in your fridge, which will help with the next strategy . . .

2. **Push your food back as you clear out the fridge:** After eating from your fridge for a few days, you'll have gone through almost half your food for the week. Moving your remaining foods back toward the airflow vents, where the temperature is colder, will help keep them fresh until the next time you food shop. This is less important if you have a duct-type airflow arrangement (see page 20), but it is crucial if you have an older fridge or a basic model with a ceiling-type airflow configuration.

3. **Moving items into the fridge:** Counter-stored items like avocados, tomatoes, and quickly ripening fruit can be brought into the fridge if needed during the week.

Food Storage Containers

"Start where you are. Use what you have. Do what you can."

—ARTHUR ASHE

Let's just say I'm a food-storage-container aficionado. And I can't stop, won't stop using our old salsa jars for storing chopped fruits and veggies, because this is major win-win territory. What you have available to you right now, today, is more important than running out to buy new things. You do not need to buy anything new to be able to start your fridge practice. In fact, I want you to decide that you're going to start with the solutions you already have at your disposal.

I save glass jars for reuse to the point that my family has nicknamed me Jar Jar Binks, or "Jar Jar" for short—a *Star Wars* reference, and one of the most-annoying-but-admittedly-fitting nicknames of all time. I have close to one hundred glass jars packed into our 1,700-square-foot home (we have the cat lady, the plant lady, and may I present *the glass jar lady*!). Many of these were saved for me by family and neighbors—my hubby literally checks with me first to see if he can go ahead and recycle his salsa jar.

You'll be amazed at what you can upcycle from your fridge and pantry right now—one of the most beautiful fridges I've ever seen was shared with me by a reader who used a bunch of old pasta sauce jars for storing chopped produce.

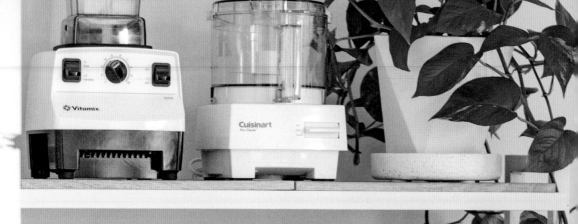

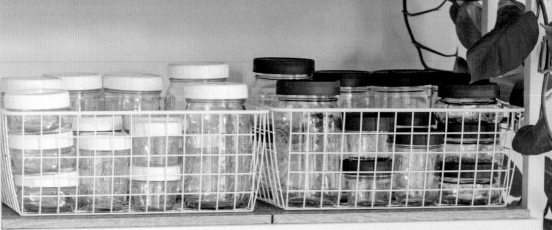

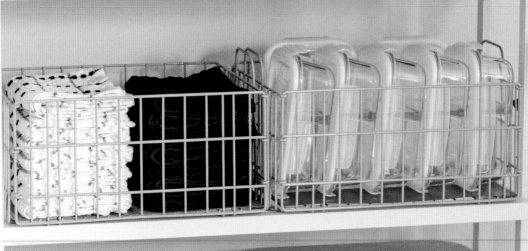

I'd much rather you made a time commitment than a monetary commitment to kick things off. Once you've proven to yourself that you're ready to take *action* toward cultivating your fridge practice, you can reward yourself by going out to get all the shiny new things!

GLASS VERSUS PLASTIC

There's one common question I'm asked when someone sees one of my fridge pics for the first time: *What food storage containers do you use?*

I consciously uncoupled with plastic food storage containers back in 2014. The reason was simple: I saw a set of glass storageware at Costco for a great price and decided to try it. That original set had about ten pieces, and I had just started exploring prepping my fridge.

I noticed a huge difference in freshness when I used those containers. Sometimes it was truly shocking. Over the next 3 years, I changed all my storage containers to glass, and I haven't looked back since.

I prefer glass containers to plastic ones because:

1. Food seems to stay fresher in glass containers.
2. Glass storage is more ecofriendly.
3. Glass storage makes reheating easier.
4. Glass doesn't leach flavors or chemicals and resists degradation.

Does Glass Really Keep Your Food Fresher for Longer?

To answer this question, I interviewed Brad W. Bolling, an assistant professor of food science at the University of Wisconsin–Madison, to find out exactly why food was lasting longer in glass than plastic. There's no peer-reviewed scientific evidence that glass performs better than plastic when it comes to shelf life and freshness, but Brad did have some insight into why I noticed such a big difference when I made the switch.

He explained that the more important factor for food freshness was actually the seal on the lids of your food storage containers; hard plastic lids with rubberized gaskets keep foods fresher longer. The thickness of the container also contributes to shelf life, so thicker plastic performs more like glass. Brad also said the differences in lids and container thickness really only make a difference in shelf life after the 5-to-7-day mark, when you're trying to extend storage to 10 or more days.

As I look back on my own experience, I now realize that much of the plastic-glass disparity I'd experienced boiled down to the fact that I was using cheap disposable plastic containers with push-down tops. If I'd been using higher-grade rigid plastic containers with tight-fitting snap-closure rubberized-gasket lids, the difference in freshness wouldn't have been as extreme.

Now, all that being said, there is one area where glass outperforms plastic, and that is when you take a chilled food container out of your fridge. Glass retains the cool temperature better than plastic containers do, which helps keep food fresher for longer. This is particularly helpful if you forget to immediately put your containers back in the fridge after you're done serving a meal.

If you happen to have an amazing set of thick, rigid-plastic food storage containers at home right now, don't toss them and go out and buy glass. Use what you've got, and bring glass storage into the fold on the periphery.

Glass Is the Ecofriendly Alternative

Plastic is terrible for the environment. Only about 9 percent of all plastic ever gets recycled, and even then, the process of breaking down and reusing plastics often leaves a heavy carbon footprint. Glass is made from naturally abundant materials that are more easily acquired than oil (the fundamental component of plastic), so the environmental impact is smaller. The glass used in almost every glass food container on the market is soda-lime glass. It's ideal for recycling because it can be softened and melted many times over, using less energy than it takes to recycle plastics.

Glass Storage Makes Reheating Easier and Safer

When foods in plastic containers are reheated in a microwave, the plastic leaches phthalates and bisphenol A (BPA), or sometimes a BPA substitute called BPS (found in some products advertised as BPA-free). These are man-made chemicals added to plastic to help it keep its shape and pliability; they are known hormone disruptors and can cause reproductive harm in adults and growth and development harm in children.

Glass Doesn't Leach Flavors and Resists Degradation

Have you ever taken a drink from a plastic water bottle and tasted the plastic? Not fun. I've often noticed a similar taste when eating food from plastic containers (more often with thinner types of plastic). Some particularly acidic foods can accelerate plastic degradation and leaching.

MY RECOMMENDED PICKS

Here are the storage containers, reusable plastic fridge bins, and accessories I use in my fridges.

Mason Jars

These are the most economical glass storage solutions—they're simple, inexpensive, and made in the USA! Used since the late 1850s for home canning and food preservation, you'll find infinite uses for mason jars in your fridge (and pretty much everywhere else in your home, too).

I always recommend that readers looking to transition to glass storage containers start with Ball brand mason jars (other great brands include Kerr and Weck, or look for generic juicing jars). To start, I recommend quart-size jars. You can pick up a set of twelve for about $30, and you'll be able to store any kind of fresh produce or cooked foods in them. After that, I suggest branching out to either half-pint or pint sizes. This will allow you to condense your food into smaller jars during the week (remember, that's a key to extending a food's shelf life—see page 44).

Wide Mouth or Regular Mouth?

I generally prefer widemouthed jars because of their ease of use—there's just more room for pouring in warm soups and compotes or larger pieces of cut produce. Regular-mouth jars work better for on-the-go-type preps like layered fruit parfaits and overnight oats, since they're usually divided into smaller portions.

I recommend getting a food funnel that corresponds to each mouth type. They are inexpensive and really keep things tidy when you're filling your jars.

When deciding on your food storage containers, you want to make them similar to the size and shape of your fridge. For example, in my side-by-side fridge I like to use taller mason jars, because there's more height between the shelves. Long storage containers work well in freezer-top standard-depth models because there's so much extra space at the back of the shelves. Squat, widemouthed jars work well in French door fridges because of the style's shallower and wider shelves.

Favorite Sizes and Uses

- **Half-pint:** Holds 1 cup. Ideal for chopped herbs, seeds, small portions of leftovers, and individual servings of overnight oats or fruit.
- **Pint:** Holds 2 cups. Ideal for portioning soups, stews, and other meals and for weekly storage of salad dressings, sauces, and other condiments, as well as dips like hummus. This is also the jar size I use most frequently for fresh herb storage.
- **Quart:** Holds 4 cups. Ideal for large portions of soup, plant milks, home-made broth, and chopped veggies.

Mason Jar Lids

- **Original tin lids:** Mason jars come with tin-plated steel lid tops and screw-on rings. These two-piece lids are intended for single use in the home canning and preserving process. Many people use them repeatedly for food storage, but because they aren't water resistant, they can be prone to rust. Each lid cover has a white undercoating to protect it from degradation from any liquid in the jar. I use these lids for dry pantry storage and when I'm prepping big batches of soups for the week. When you add warm food to the jar and cover it immediately with the lid, the lid top forms a suction seal. Use caution when later opening the lids, as the seal can stick and make it difficult to pull the lid top off the jar (I like to use a dish towel to protect my fingers when breaking the seal).
- **White plastic lids:** These are the lids I use most often for foods that I'm handling every day (sauces, dressings, hummus, chopped produce). They're

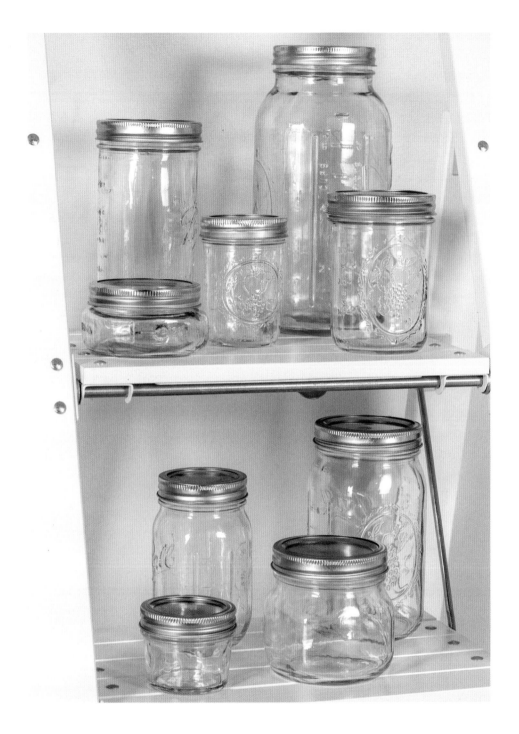

easier to use than the two-piece tin lids, and you don't have to worry about rust. Some readers have reported leakage issues with these lids. I use mine for jars that are upright in the fridge, so they've worked fine for me. I use Ball brand, but you can find a variety of brands of similar lids at Target and Walmart or online.

- **Leakproof black plastic lids:** These lids are made from a thicker plastic than the white lids and don't have reported leaking issues.

Glass Snap-Lock Storage Sets

If you're looking to invest in your food storage solutions, glass storage sets should be next on your list. What sets these containers apart is the thickness of the glass (great for temperature retention) and the fact that they are shatter-proof, can be used in the oven (without the lids!), and freeze wonderfully.

This is a great option if your goal after reading this book is to start doing more meal prepping. The tightness and fit of the snap-lock lids make all the difference in freshness. I prefer hard plastic lids to soft rubber lids. The two brands I use and recommend are Pyrex and Glasslock. Made in the US and Korea, respectively, my original sets from each of these brands have lasted me over six years (with very frequent use), and they're still going strong!

Remember when we talked about the importance of a hard-plastic snap-lock rubberized-gasket lid (page 48)? That's why these two brands stand out when it comes to food freshness. The lids don't lose their hold over time like other brands I've tried.

I recommend starting with a ten-piece set (including lids) and growing your collection from there. These sets are pricier when you buy online, but I see them on sale frequently at Costco and sometimes at Target and Walmart.

Sectioned Glass Containers

There are two types of people in this world: those who don't mind their foods touching and those who do! I recently bought a set of sectioned containers from a brand called Prep Naturals after I saw a fellow food blogger raving about them for meal prep. They're made with thick glass and come with snap-lock lids. These are a great choice if you're looking for something less pricey than the glass sets I recommended above and you intend to use them for meal prepping. Pyrex has also released a new line of sectioned glass containers that would be a great choice, too.

Fridge Bins and Trays

Fridge bins and trays help you create zones in your fridge (I give some examples of zone types in the fridge "case studies," starting on page 69). Bins can also help you use more of the space toward the back of your fridge; they work as a kind of drawer that you can pull out to easily access items stored at the back, without knocking over everything in front in the process. You can arrange items inside the bins so you can see everything at a glance from above.

They're great for containing multiple mason jars—you can pull out the whole bin and have all your components (for your in-fridge salad bar, for example; see page 174) in one place.

Which Bins/Trays Should I Buy?

Buy bins and trays that help you utilize unused space in your fridge. This might mean deeper bins for standard-depth fridges and stackable bins to take advantage of vertical space. Avoid bins and drawers that are bulky and reduce your actual storage space—I know these look really appealing, but in my experience, they aren't maximizing space.

If you have a lot of loose bags (salad mixes, baby carrots) and/or small items (yogurts, condiments spilling over from door storage, snacks), investing in bins is a great way to quickly rein in the chaos.

What about "specialty" bins? For example, bins for your eggs or sodas. You have to decide if this will help you free up space in your fridge or if it's just going to look good. In my experience, egg bins look amazing but take up much more space than a normal egg carton.

Remember, bins alone are not going to keep uncovered produce fresh, even covered stackable bins (air makes its way in through the loose lid and handle opening). Uncovered leafy produce will immediately wilt, while thick-skinned produce (like bell preppers and cucumbers) will last a day or two at most. You always want to cover raw produce with plastic or keep it in an airtight

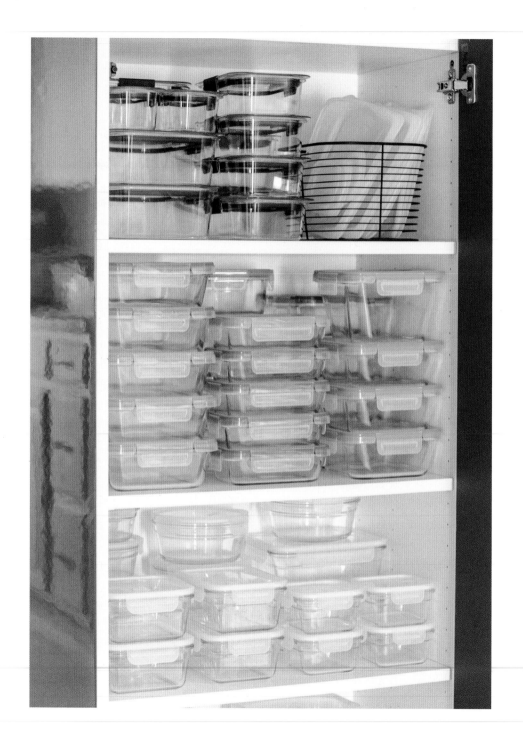

container to prevent moisture loss from the cool, dry air produced by your refrigerator.

- **Standard-depth freezer-top recommendations:** I like to use two 12 by 14-inch, 1½-inch-deep trays to create a drawerlike function to make items at the back of the shelves easier to reach. And since this is where I like to store meats and dairy, it helps prevent any spills from spreading to lower shelves. Stackable bins work on the middle shelf to help utilize vertical space. I like using 16 by 9-inch metal wire baskets on the top shelf in the freezer section, as they act as drawers to store boxes and bags of frozen foods.
- **Counter-depth side-by-side recommendations:** Because shelves are not as deep in this model, I like to use 10-inch-deep stackable bins in the fresh and freezer sections to utilize vertical space.
- **Counter-depth French door recommendations:** I use 12½-inch-deep bins on the upper and middle shelves and 14½-inch-deep bins on the sides of the lower shelf. Measure your model's shelves to make sure the same dimensions work (especially on the lower shelf).
- **Plastic:** Reusable plastic bins are lightweight; I've had my set for years now and use them daily.
- **Metal:** If you want as much plastic out of your life as possible, metal wire or mesh storage baskets are a great way to go. I happen to think they look quite stylish, too.
- **Natural fibers:** Natural-fiber baskets may be less practical for use inside your fridge because they are susceptible to damage from moisture and spills. But as long as you give them a check during your weekly wipe downs, they can be a great fridge organization tool, especially if you already have them available in another area of your home.

Lazy Susans

If you have a lot of condiments—more than can fit in your door storage—arranging them on a lazy Susan is a great organization strategy. This minimizes spills because you're not constantly reaching over other items. Lazy Susans also work well for the smaller shelves in side-by-side fridges.

ECOFRIENDLY FRIDGE STORAGE SOLUTIONS

Many of the recommendations I've given so far would work in a zero-waste fridge. But when you're approaching your fridge with this goal, I think it's important to start by thinking about what you can *reuse* first. Hit up your recycling bin before heading to the store. Pasta sauce jars, condiment jars, jelly jars—all these can be cleaned and used again to store healthful foods in your fridge!

To remove sticky labels and stamps: It's a good idea to gather at least five or six jars and do them all at one time. Put the jars in your sink and fill with hot water till you've just covered the jars. Let them soak for about 10 minutes. Drain the sink and begin peeling off the paper or plastic labels. I use a spoon to help scratch off any particularly resistant labels. Once you've removed the labels, you will usually be left with opaque lines of glue. Dip a Q-tip in rubbing alcohol and apply liberally to the glue strips. Use a razor (or that spoon again, with some extra elbow grease) to scrape off the glue. Some glues are extra stubborn, and in a few cases I've had to use an adhesive remover. I recommend Duck brand adhesive remover, which comes with a built-in scraper on top of the cap (model 527263, 5.45 ounce bottle). You don't need to use much—just enough to dampen the glue residue.

If the jar has a "use by" stamp on it, you can usually get those off with a Q-tip dipped in rubbing alcohol. Sometimes these dates are stamped on the jar lid; I've found these don't come off as well as those on the glass itself. Unfortunately, not all stamps will come off, but it's worth trying.

Alternatives to Plastic Wrap and Plastic Bags

- **Dish towels:** Wrapping leafy greens in natural cloth (like a cotton or linen dish towel) is a great way to keep them fresh and prevent wilting. This method is great for striking that delicate balance between adequate and excessive moisture. Draping towels over pots and jars (after the food has cooled) can also do the trick (and actually *did* the trick for many years before plastic wrap was ever invented).

- **Cloth produce bags:** Bags made with natural fibers like linen, cotton, or bamboo are an ecofriendly alternative to plastic produce bags from the

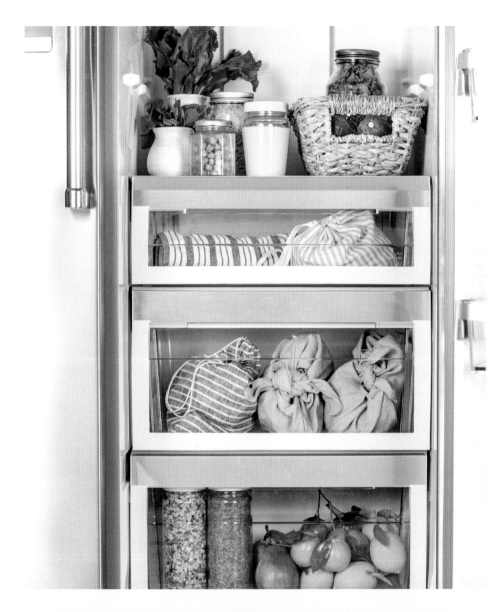

When using cotton or linen storage solutions, you want to make sure there is initial and sustained moisture. You can rinse your produce before placing it in the bags or run the material under cool water and wring out well before adding the produce. Make sure to keep the fabric moist with quick spritzes every 2 to 3 days, or when it's dry to the touch.

grocery store. I especially love the linen greens bag I found on Etsy; you spray it with water to create that humid environment that greens love.

- **Cloth bowl covers:** Usually made of linen, cotton, or laminated cotton, these circular pieces of material with elasticized edges fit snugly over bowls.
- **Beeswax wraps:** A great alternative to plastic wrap, these reusable wraps are made from cotton cloth infused with beeswax, and can be molded around food or over bowls. (Note that these are not a vegan product.)
- **Dutch ovens and other lidded cookware:** If you have the space, just go ahead and put the whole pot in the fridge (be sure it's fully cooled first, though, or you risk humidity problems). This method works well if you'll be eating the food in the next 2 days.
- **Silicone bags:** These thick, high-quality silicone bags with tight seals are a reusable alternative to zip-top plastic bags.
- **Ceramic dinner plates:** This is a wonderful low-tech way to cover a bowl of food before storing in the fridge.
- **Ceramic and silicone and glass reusable to-go containers:** Take your food on the go with W&P brand "Porter" to-go containers, which are made with ecofriendlier materials like ceramic and glass coated in silicone.
- **Silicone stretch lids:** These come in varying sizes and work like plastic wrap. They can go over bowls or over sliced produce (like a lemon, avocado, or fruit).
- **Vintage glass refrigerator dishes:** Although the seal isn't airtight, these containers have lasted for decades and can be a great ecofriendly alternative to buying newly manufactured sets. Look for dishes stamped with Corning, Pyrex, and Anchor Hocking.

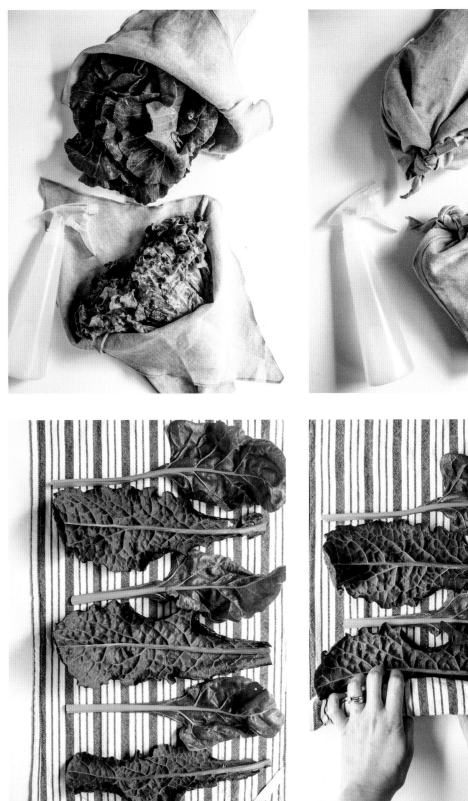
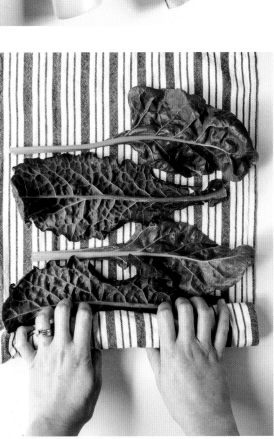

How to Organize by Fridge Type

One reaction I hear from readers over and over again is "I can't do that because I don't own a French door fridge." I'm here to tell you that no matter what type of fridge you own, you *can* organize it to work for you!

FREEZER-TOP

Freezer-top fridges typically allocate 75 percent of their total storage space to fresh food and 25 percent to frozen foods. The fridge shelves are boxy and deep, with most standard-depth models running about 29 inches deep and 29 inches wide.

You have a lot of space for fresh food storage in this configuration. You won't be able to keep everything at eye level, but what it lacks in this area it makes up for with its extra shelf depth.

Top shelf: If you have a basic, ceiling-type airflow configuration, you'll notice that the top shelf is the coolest. I like to keep dairy beverages, meat, eggs, and homemade sauces and condiments on this shelf, no more than three containers deep—this allows ample space for airflow so the cooled air from the freezer makes it down the back of the fridge to the lower shelves. Prepped soups or meals that you want to eat later in the week do wonderfully toward the back on this shelf, as this is the coldest spot in the fridge.

Middle shelf: The next shelf down is ideal for beverages, yogurts, cooked whole grains, and chopped fruits and veggies. Make sure to leave at least 4 inches of space from the back wall to ensure air continues to flow downward.

Deli drawer: I don't like the placement of the deli drawer in this fridge type (mine sits under the top shelf), and functionally, I find it very awkward to use. Instead, I use a shallow plastic fridge container to house animal products that need to stay the coldest, including cheeses, eggs, raw meat, and deli meats, and store the container on the top shelf.

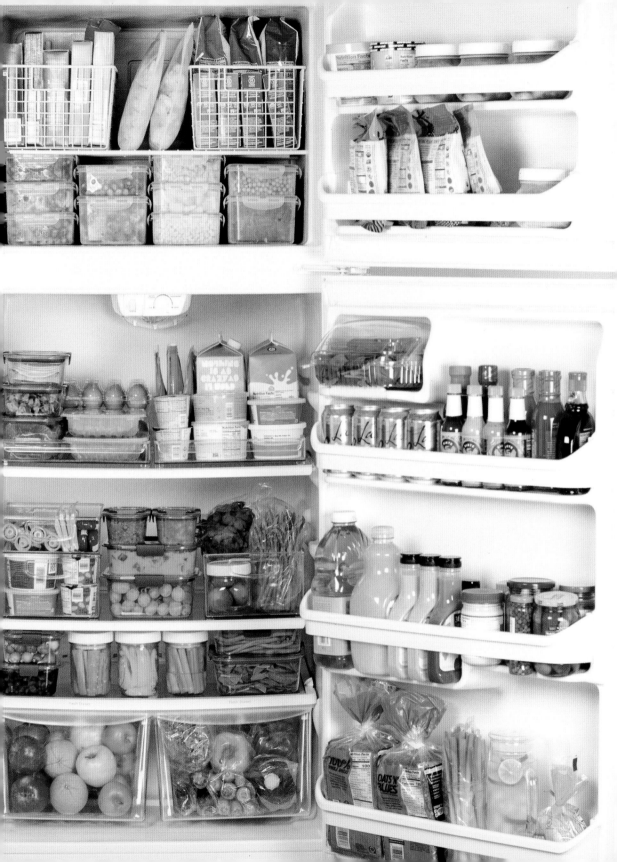

Bottom shelf: The shelf above the crisper drawer is ideal for storing lettuces and leafy greens (if you're not storing them in the crisper). This level is also ideal for bulk pantry items such as flours, nuts, and seeds. (Yes, you can refrigerate those! See page 150.) Be careful not to inadvertently cover the 2.5-inch grill along the back of the shelf, as this is the predominant source of air for the crisper bins.

Crisper drawers: The deep crisper bins on this unit work particularly well for long-term fruit storage, especially for citrus fruits and apples (though these are best stored separately, if you're looking to keep them for longer than 2 weeks).

Door: Door storage on basic, ceiling-type airflow models can be a warm spot. I recommend storing fresh herbs, breads, flours, or spices and store-bought condiments in this area.

Freezer: The freezer is the most important place to keep organized in this refrigerator type—especially when you have a basic, lower-priced model—

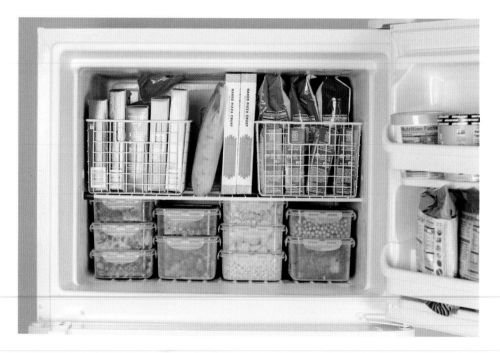

because there's only one source of airflow from the freezer down into the refrigerated compartment. That airflow has to be powerful enough to make it all the way down to each shelf in the refrigerator without the aid of extra nozzles, so if you have a freezer-top fridge, *it's critical not to overfill or stuff your freezer*. Leave at least 3 inches, preferably 4, between your food and the back wall of the freezer compartment.

Store-bought bags of frozen foods (like fruits, veggies, chicken strips, and french fries) tend to get pushed back and can interfere with the evaporator airflow on the back wall of the freezer compartment. I recommend corralling bags and small containers of frozen foods in rigid plastic bins or trays that you can easily move away from the back wall to help you maintain that essential space for airflow.

Note that if you have a newer (2016 or later), higher-end freezer-top model, you may have a dual evaporator configuration, which means you'll only need to leave about 2 inches from the back wall empty for adequate airflow.

SIDE-BY-SIDE

Side-by-side fridges are designed to maximize freezer capacity, with about 60 percent of their total storage space allotted to fresh food and 40 percent to frozen foods. The fridge and freezer shelves are boxy and shallow, with most counter-depth models running at about 13 inches deep and 17.5 inches wide.

Most side-by-side fridge units on the market today have a duct-type airflow configuration. This is great news, because it ensures ideal airflow to every shelf in the refrigerated compartment, meaning you don't have to worry about warm or cold areas as much. (The only exception to this is if you live in a humid climate, in which case the areas near the doors may trend warmer than the rest of the compartment.)

Properly stored foods can live happily on every shelf in a duct-type side-by-side fridge, and you don't need to worry about placing items too far toward the back of the shelves. So instead of breaking things down shelf by shelf, I suggest using these strategies:

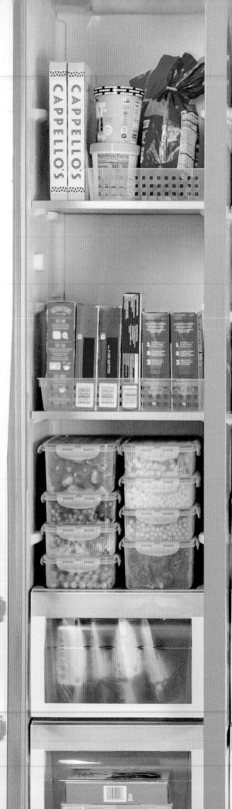
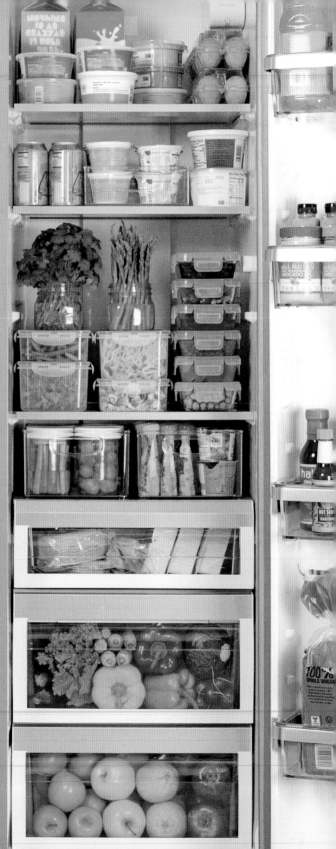

Put your best food forward: I love that a side-by-side model allows you to store food at eye level in both the fresh and frozen compartments. Take maximum advantage of this design aspect by placing those foods that are most important for your healthy lifestyle at the front of the fridge, where you will see them. Keep long-storage items toward the bottom half of each compartment and frequently used items in the upper half. One thing worth mentioning: From a food safety standpoint, it's best to store raw meat on a lower shelf to avoid contaminating other foods with dripping juices; in this configuration, I store meat in the deli drawer under the lowest shelf. But keeping meats in a fridge bin can also do the trick for containing possible drippings.

Create themed zones: Delegating shelves by theme can also be a helpful organization strategy. For example, I have a shelf completely dedicated to my in-fridge salad bar (see page 174), the components for which are housed in a large, flat bin so I can easily pull out everything at once. If you have small kids, store kid-friendly snacks such as hummus, veggies, and fruit on the lower shelves where kids can reach them.

Freezer: The freezer in a side-by-side unit can be challenging to organize because of the tall, narrow shelves. It's tempting to stack items or bags in these areas, only for them to subsequently fall out. I recommend using a mix of stackable rigid plastic storage containers and bins to keep bags of frozen food secure. When I can, I also like to keep one shelf reserved for freezing in-season fresh produce for long-term storage (see page 141).

> Think about how you actually want to use your freezer, and then make room for the functionality you want by getting rid of the things that don't serve your goals. For example, if reducing food waste is important to you, then having a space for veggie scrap collection will serve you better than storing a huge chicken breast you may not eat for some time. Conversely, if you're trying to stretch your grocery budget by buying things in bulk when they're on sale, you might prioritize those items in your freezer at the expense of extra space for storing scraps or freezing produce.

FRENCH DOOR

French door fridges are designed to maximize the accessibility of fresh foods. They typically devote 70 percent of their total storage space to fresh foods and 30 percent to frozen foods. The fridge shelves are long and rectangular, with most counter-depth models running about 13.5 inches deep and 33.5 inches wide. A French door fridge truly acts as a fresh-foods showcase because the whole refrigerated compartment is at eye level. I can't tell you how nice this is for a tall girl like me.

Duct-type airflow configurations are standard in most French door fridge units, with many newer models (2016 and later) having dual evaporators as another upgraded standard feature. These fridges are constantly working to keep air moving at the right temperature, with sensors placed throughout the refrigerated compartment. As a result, I've noticed they tend to run a bit colder than their temperature setting indicates.

Top shelf: In my first year of owning my French door model fridge, a lot of my food, especially on the top shelf, was inadvertently frozen because of the more advanced cooling technology. Now I typically keep homemade sauces and condiments on the top shelf, pulling all the containers as far forward as possible to minimize freezing.

Middle shelf: This is where I like to keep my prepared food for the week, such as cooked whole grains and individually portioned meals. I also like to keep some chopped fruits on this shelf so they're in view and easily accessible.

Bottom shelf: I look at this shelf as an extension of my crisper drawers. It's where I keep prepped salad greens and chopped veggies.

Crisper drawers: I keep my most frequently used nuts and seeds, whole fresh fruits, and tofu in the crisper drawers.

Bottom drawer: The best place for deli meats and cheeses.

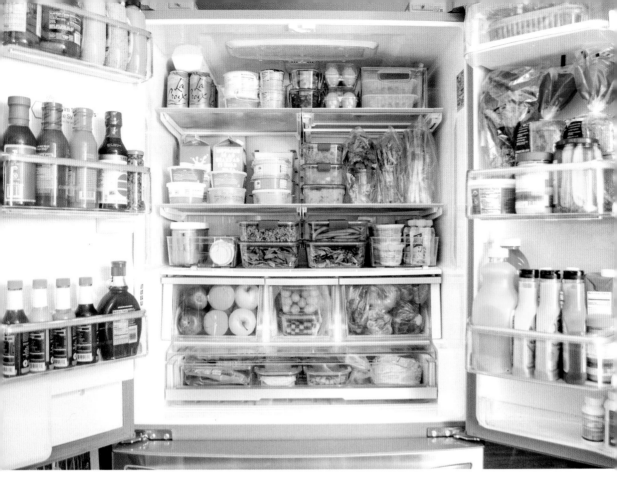

Door storage: Because of the duct-type airflow and added temperature sensors in these models, door storage is just as temperature regulated as the rest of the fridge, and as long as you're not an excessive door opener (more than the average fifteen to twenty times per day), you should have no problem with foods stored on the doors.

Freezer: Most French door fridge models come with a pull-out drawer-style freezer. Some newer models continue the French doors on the bottom freezer portion of the unit, with pull-out drawers within.

My pull-out freezer has three interior drawers. In the shallower top drawer, I like to use long, narrow plastic bins to store frozen meats for my family (burgers, hot dogs, roasts, and loin cuts). I also keep ice creams here.

The middle drawer is the shallowest and is perfect for freezing fresh berries, banana slices, or peak-season produce you want to stock up on at great prices. This can be as easy as lining a baking sheet with parchment paper and laying the produce on top. I'll also keep shallow tubs of frozen fruits and veggies in this drawer so they stay top of mind for everyday use.

The bottom drawer is the deepest and typically comes with a built-in divider. I've found this drawer works best for bags and boxed items (like frozen pizzas). I like to "file" our bags of frozen food so I can look into the drawer and get a bird's-eye view of what we have on hand.

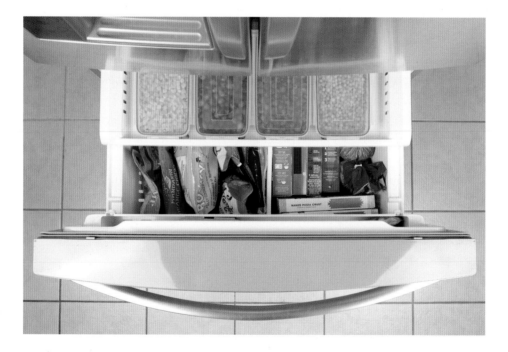

FRIDGE CASE STUDIES

Your life situation is going to dictate how you organize your fridge and how you prioritize what you put inside. The way you use your fridge will change depending on where you are in your life. Let's cover some strategies that are helpful for each stage.

Dorm/Mini Fridge

The biggest concern I hear from readers is how can they get maximum fresh, healthy foods in such a small space. As a general rule, you want to prioritize your space. So, instead of loading your fridge with beverages, have a designated space that you can refill daily and free up that space for fresh produce instead. Keep in mind that shelf life is going to be reduced in a mini fridge (especially basic models) because of temperature fluctuations from opening the fridge doors. There's very little room in a mini fridge, and when you open the door, the cool air escapes and warm air is let in. Keep prepped produce pushed back in the main compartment to keep a more consistent temperature, and use door storage for beverages and whole fruits like citrus and apples.

- Buy precut fresh veggies to serve with hummus or guacamole (see Easy Veggie Cups, page 167, and Easy Fruit Cups, page 168).
- Cut broccoli and cauliflower have a long shelf life and are great eaten cold or flash-steamed in the microwave.
- Baby spinach has a long shelf life and works as a quick salad base.
- Overnight Oats (pages 209–213) and Chia Puddings (pages 217–221) can be a quick healthy breakfast or cure a sweet tooth straight out of the fridge.

Roommates

Sharing your fridge with roommates is a challenge, and much will be dependent on how well you know each other starting out.

- **Color-Coded Storage:** I'm not a big fan of designating entire fridge shelves to each roommate because, as we've learned, there are cooler and warmer zones of the fridge. Instead, commit each roommate to a certain color. You can find plastic storage bins in different colors (the dollar store is great for this) and different color mason jar lids can be bought in bulk on Amazon.

- **Separating Shelves:** Use masking tape to carve out space on each major shelf, and use stackable storage containers and bins to utilize vertical space.

- **Labeling:** If you choose this approach, it's a great idea to have a magnetized holder on your fridge for masking tape or labels and a Sharpie. Label whole bins for each roommate, and then have a communal shelf where you can label leftovers or preps for the week.

- **3-Way Deli Drawer:** Use a plastic desk organizer (Sterlite makes a 3-drawer model) to add more drawer space that is easily divided.

- **Communal Condiments:** Make an agreement with your roommates early on about sharing certain key condiments like ketchup, mayo, mustard, and pickles and storing these items on the door. This saves you room in the key fridge storage areas by avoiding duplicates. Start by having each roommate pitch in for a condiment haul and then replenish at a set interval.

Singles and Young Couples

You're in an ideal situation here where much of how you approach organizing and stocking your refrigerator will come down to your personal eating intentions. Use the fridge goals we identified at the beginning of the book to guide your approach.

- **Dietary Differences:** I've had quite a few readers reach out to me about sharing their fridge with a significant other who eats differently than they do. For some this can be a health difference, for others a moral difference. Focus your fridge on what you do have in common. Then create safe spaces for each other using opaque bins or designating entire drawers.

Families with Babies and Toddlers

The key concern I hear from these kinds of readers is how to organize the fridge to save time with an emphasis on providing healthy food for their growing kids.

- **Newborn-Specific Zones:** Just like the rest of the house, when baby arrives, they're going to take up space in the fridge. Designate a bin in the fridge or freezer for premade bottles and/or frozen breast milk. Leftovers will be more important than ever as you look for quick ways to reheat and eat.

- **Solid Foods:** Create a dedicated zone in the freezer for freezing homemade baby food, if you make your own. It felt like from ages 1 to 5 all I did was make my kids snacks. Have a designated bin in the fridge for cut fruit and veggies that you can quickly pull out for healthy snacks.
- **Dinner Bin:** After the survival mode that is the first 3 to 6 months with an infant at home, you're likely looking to start focusing on your health again. Make a designated dinner bin where you can quickly round up all the ingredients you need to make dinner later.
- **Leftovers:** Toddlers are notoriously finnicky eaters, and saving untouched snacks and meals is a must to protect your sanity and cut down on time in the kitchen. You want to reserve ample space in your fridge for leftovers. Use two clear fridge bins to separate grown-up leftovers from the kids'.

Families with Elementary School-Age Kids

At this stage, family schedules are getting busier and kids are becoming more independent.

- **Lunch Box Station:** Designate a fridge bin to all the ingredients you need to make weekday lunches. You or your older kid can easily grab the bin in the morning and have everything they need to make a healthy lunch and take-to-school snacks. This was also helpful for us during the pandemic stay-at-home period, when the kids often made their own lunches.
- **Independent Snacking:** Labelling and bins can be very helpful here so your kids aren't rummaging through the fridge looking for their stuff and calling for Mom to come find their Go-Gurts. Remember that your kids will eat only the snacks available to them, so if getting healthier is a top priority, fill your snack bins with what you want them to be eating.

Families with Teenagers and Young Adults

Your fridge is going to be opened up a lot more during this life stage as teenagers are notorious boredom eaters with seemingly endless appetites. The key consideration with this increased use is to minimize the amount of time your fridge doors are open (this affects food shelf life and how often your fridge is running).

- **Favorites Bins:** There's nothing teens love more than autonomy, so designate a bin for their personal favorite foods that is easy to find and pull out of the fridge. Put drinks, snacks, and meals all in the same bin so they don't have to go back and forth.
- **Young Adults:** Use some of the guidance on pages 69–70 for roommates to help ease the tension around fridge sharing.
- **Defining Standards:** I hear from a lot of frustrated readers who are sick of their teens and young adults trashing the fridge. Sit down together and come up with a system using the principles in this book then see if it helps. Keep adjusting weekly until you get to a place where everyone is on board with keeping up minimum family fridge standards.

Empty Nesters and Retired Couples

Your fridge is yours again, and the possibilities are endless! If you're retired now, you may have more time to dedicate to on-demand cooking, and your fridge can transition to a source of culinary inspiration.

- **Budgeting:** Decide on your eating goals, grocery budget, and how often you want to go to the store. If you have more time to dedicate to shopping you don't need things to last so long in the fridge.
- **Notes on Storage Containers:** The biggest feedback I get from older readers is how heavy and hard to open food storage containers can be. Keep this in mind when deciding on your fridge storage. Glass containers may look pretty, but they are certainly heavy. And some sets of plastic containers with tight-fitting lids can be very hard to handle. You may have to sacrifice a bit of shelf life for ease of use.

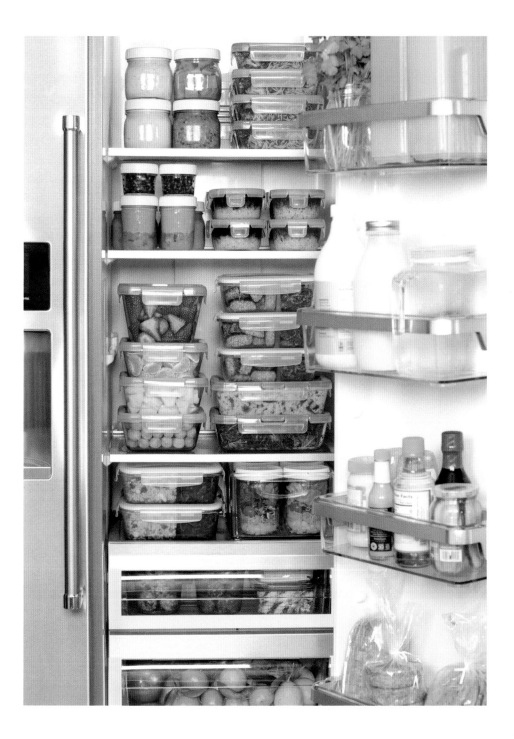

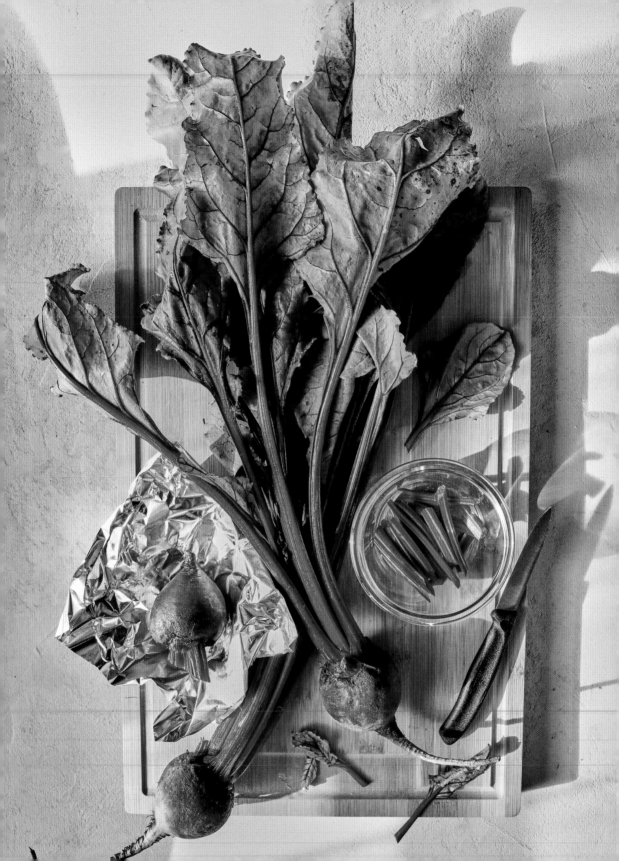

Part 3

THE PRODUCE PREP AND STORAGE GUIDE

According to appliance maker LG, the average US household wastes an average of $1,800 worth of food each year because it goes bad in the fridge. Produce accounts for a big chunk of that—we've all regretfully tossed out some yellowed salad greens or past-their-prime apples at some point. Because eating fresh fruits and veggies is so important to a healthy lifestyle, and because maximizing their shelf life is a big key to reducing food waste, I've created this guide to help you get the most out of your produce. Flip to the page for any particular vegetable, fruit, or herb and learn everything you need to know on how to process and store it, as well as how long you can expect it to keep, whether fresh or cooked, in some cases.

Warm and Cold Zones in Your Fridge

Beware of blanket fridge-storage advice that lumps together all types of fridges and all kinds of ambient conditions. Statements like "You should never store your eggs or milk in door storage" are just flat-out wrong in certain circumstances. We covered all the fine detail earlier in the book, but here are some highlights to remember:

- Doors are generally warmer areas of your fridge (especially if you have frequent fridge use, struggle with ambient heat and/or humidity, and/or have a more basic-model fridge).
- Crisper drawers are warmer (or can be made warmer by adjusting the sliders to allow more or less airflow).
- The back spine of the fridge is colder in back wall– and ceiling-type airflow fridges.
- In a freezer-top basic-model fridge, the back of the top shelf is the coldest area. Lower shelves have less direct airflow, so they are not as cold.
- Duct-type airflow fridges give the most consistent temperature because they have many added sensors throughout the unit. You have the most freedom with this type of fridge. I've stored eggs and dairy milk in the door sections and never had a problem.
- Door storage is a great place to keep your herbs (covered in plastic or tented in a glass jar) because the temperature is generally warmer and more humid—especially in basic-model, ceiling-type airflow fridges.

Produce Storage

How long will a given piece of produce last in the fridge? The answer, unfortunately, is *it depends*: It depends on your particular fridge (its age and effectiveness) and the climate where you live, as well as the age of the produce and how it was handled before you even brought it home.

This guide shares the science behind produce shelf life and the storage techniques I've found work best.

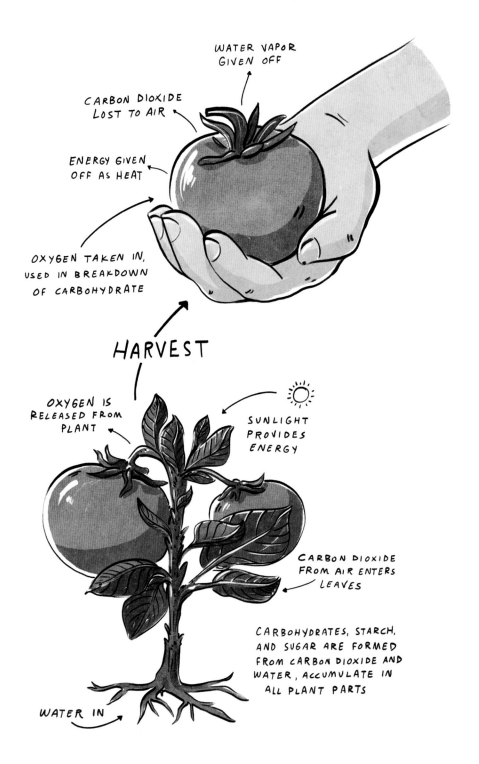

WATER VAPOR GIVEN OFF

CARBON DIOXIDE LOST TO AIR

ENERGY GIVEN OFF AS HEAT

OXYGEN TAKEN IN, USED IN BREAKDOWN OF CARBOHYDRATE

HARVEST

OXYGEN IS RELEASED FROM PLANT

SUNLIGHT PROVIDES ENERGY

CARBON DIOXIDE FROM AIR ENTERS LEAVES

CARBOHYDRATES, STARCH, AND SUGAR ARE FORMED FROM CARBON DIOXIDE AND WATER, ACCUMULATE IN ALL PLANT PARTS

WATER IN

The temperature and humidity recommendations I give in this section are based on commercially used data that is meant to inform conditions during cold-chain transit. But industrial produce distributors are able to set storage rooms to exact recommended temperatures and humidity levels in a way you likely can't reproduce in your home kitchen. Nevertheless, I still find this information helpful—these optimal temperature and humidity ranges can give you some insight into how your environment compares to the absolute best conditions for any particular type of produce.

THE LIFE CYCLE OF PRODUCE

When a plant is growing, it's building up carbohydrates using water from its roots, carbon dioxide from the air, and sunlight in a process we all know as photosynthesis. The amazing by-product of this process is oxygen, which the plant releases into the air.

When that plant's produce is harvested, the cycle reverses. All the carbohydrates the plant so diligently built up begin the process of breaking down. Oxygen is taken in from the surrounding air and breaks down the stored carbohydrates into carbon dioxide and water. During this reverse process, the produce releases water vapor, heat, and carbon dioxide into the air.

Things to remember about fresh produce:

- It's alive.
- It breathes (a process called respiration).
- It releases heat.
- It loses moisture.
- It can get sick (from microorganisms).
- It will die (even if you do everything perfectly, the internal structure will decay over time).

UNDERSTANDING FRESHNESS FACTORS

There's a small window between when produce has reached its peak ripeness (this is usually the point where the most nutrients have accumulated) and when it's consumed. Our goal is to elongate this window as much as possible.

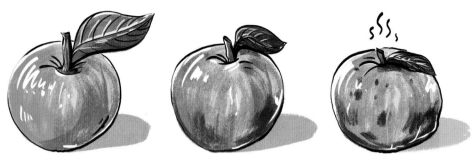

ALIVE   BREATHES   RELEASES HEAT

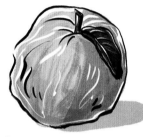
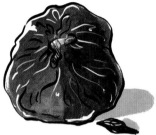
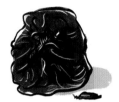

LOSES MOISTURE   CAN GET SICK   CAN EVEN DIE

There are ten factors that affect the shelf life of your produce:

1. **Temperature:** When produce is stored in a cold environment, the other nine freshness factors can't cause as much damage; things like respiration and microorganism activity are slowed down. The inverse is true as well. If your produce is stored in warm conditions, that extra heat speeds up the life cycle and accelerates produce death and decay.

2. **Humidity:** Fresh produce has an incredibly high water content. The minute a piece of fruit or a vegetable is harvested and cut off from its water supply (the plant's roots), it begins to lose water from respiration. The dry, cool air inside a refrigerator (outside the crisper drawers) is not optimal for most fresh produce. Storing your produce in a humid environment prevents moisture loss, the number one reason produce wilts and wrinkles.

3. **Respiration:** Since produce is still alive after it's harvested, it also continues to breathe. Respiration is the process of the plant breathing in oxygen from the air around it, breaking down its stored carbohydrates, and

releasing heat, water, and carbon dioxide. The warmer the temperature, the more rapid this breathing becomes. Each type of produce has its own rate of respiration and optimal storage temperature to decrease that rate.

4. **Water:** Yes, plants do need some humidity, but *excess* water can be a damaging factor. It can contribute to the degradation of the plant wall structure (think soggy greens) and be an entry point for microorganisms. The goal is to find the ideal level of moisture.

5. **Oxygen:** The more oxygen around your produce, the faster the respiration rate. When you place produce in an airtight container, you're effectively capping the amount of oxygen available for the produce to "breathe in." Since we're trying to slow down that breathing, it's important to take whatever produce you need from its storage container and then quickly cover the container again to minimize oxygen exposure.

6. **Mechanical damage:** Mechanical damage is external damage to the produce, such as bruising or piercing of the skin, that leaves produce more susceptible to microorganisms. It usually happens during harvesting or transport. At home, it can also be the result of cutting produce with a dull knife—the sharper the knife, the better for your produce, especially when you're chopping raw produce for the week.

7. **Microorganisms:** Microorganisms include mold, yeast, bacteria, and viruses. Produce is grown on farms, so it's exposed to organisms in the soil, air, and dust that gets kicked up during the growing process. Produce can be exposed to another set of microorganisms during transit and storage. Refrigeration slows down the growth of microorganisms, but it's important to know that it doesn't kill them (cooking to 165°F is a kill step). Washing helps remove most microorganisms, but not all.

8. **Chemicals in the environment:** Chemicals in the air surrounding the produce can accelerate its degradation. One of the most notable of these is ethylene, a ripening molecule released naturally by some types of produce. Fruits and vegetables can either be ethylene producers or ethylene absorbers. These are incompatible; I've noted combinations that shouldn't be stored together in the following section. Another concern here is carbon dioxide that the produce is respiring. The less air in a container, the less opportunity for respiration, creating less carbon dioxide.

9. **Light exposure:** Light activates the pores in plants (which allow gases to enter and be released by the plant). When harvested fresh produce is exposed to light (think produce at an outdoor farmers' market or located near windows in a grocery store), respiration increases and photosynthesis reactivates. This isn't a major factor for produce refrigerated at home, since our fridges are dark when they're closed, but it can be a factor in a retail setting, where produce may be stored near a source of natural or artificial light. Be mindful of farmers' market produce that has been out in the sun for a prolonged time (3 to 4 hours), and simply eat it sooner.

10. **Plant structure and enzymes:** Your produce can still "die of natural causes." If you were to keep your produce in the exact ideal conditions (effectively managing the other freshness factors) and any microorganisms were killed off (not present to begin with), it would still naturally break down. It would continue to use up its carbohydrate stores, depleting its energy and causing its structure to deteriorate, and then start to ferment due to its natural enzymes. Its pigment would change and its volume would shrink. In the end, we would see brown spots or wrinkling, signs that the produce is no longer able to maintain its cell walls properly, and ultimately, it would turn to mush. That's the point of natural decay.

FINAL FRESHNESS THOUGHTS

Probably the most frustrating thing about produce shelf life is that when you buy a piece of produce, you don't know where it falls on the spectrum of freshness—produce may be alive, but it can't tell us what it's been through.

You could be shopping at a local produce stand or farmers' market, where it's been a few short hours since harvest, or you could be shopping at a supermarket, where the produce has been shipped from all over the world. You don't know if there were gaps in the cold chain that affected temperature or humidity or if the produce was exposed to excess light at that roadside stand.

These sourcing differences will affect the overall shelf life of your produce, but it's impractical to account for every nuance. Your best judgment, combined with the guidance beginning on the next page, will help you get as much time from your produce as possible.

How to Store Your Produce
(and a Few Other Foods, Too!): Best Practices

A Few Helpful Notes

Ambient conditions: About one-third of the produce we'll cover in this section of the book is best stored in ambient conditions—meaning outside of the fridge, usually on a countertop or in a cool, dry spot. Your ambient conditions will be influenced by the climate where you live, the time of year, and the temperature in your home. If the optimal storage recommendations for a particular type of produce aren't feasible for you, just go ahead and store it in your fridge (I'll provide guidance on that, too).

Container density: When I give guidelines for filling glass containers, I may specify loosely packing or tightly packing your containers. If I don't specify, aim for the middle of the road.

Produce tenting: There are a few types of produce, like soft fresh herbs and root veggies, that I recommend storing upright in glass jars filled halfway with water, with their tops covered loosely with a plastic bag. The water creates optimal humidity conditions, the plastic protects the leaves from the fridge's cold airflow, and standing the produce upright reduces the chance of excess moisture pooling and causing leaves to slime.

Plastic bag alternatives: I'm not going to lie, plastic produce bags, especially the thicker, clear kind they often have at farmers' markets, are one of the best tools for maximizing whole produce storage times. Unfortunately, they are downright rotten for our environment. I make it a practice to wash out and reuse these bags as often as possible. Please note that food-safe silicone bags can always be used in place of plastic, and they have almost identical shelf-life compatibility! I also provide storage guidance for ecofriendly cotton and linen produce bags.

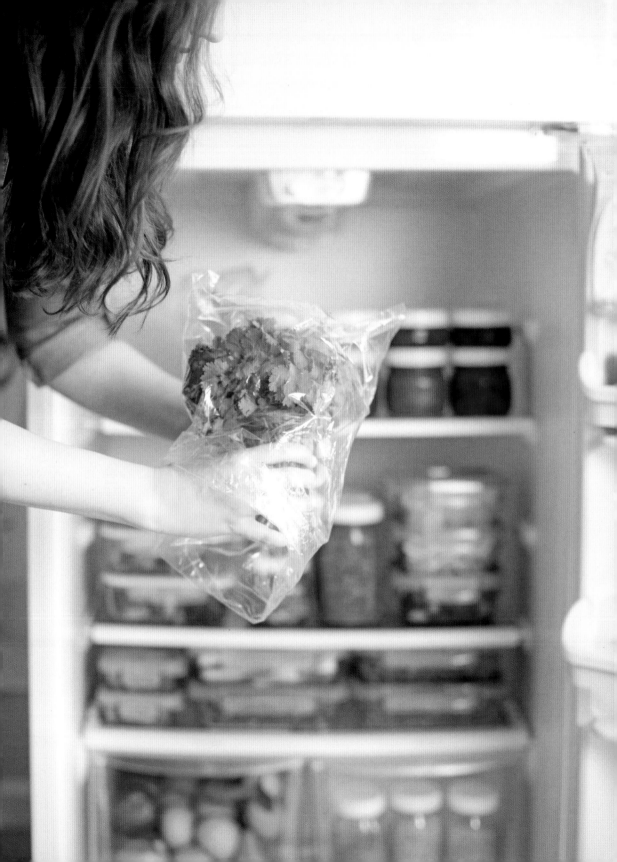

HOW TO TEND YOUR FRIDGE

I give a range of storage times for most items in this section. So what is going to get you from the low end of my recommended shelf life to the maximum? Some things, as we've already learned, are out of your control. Like how fresh the produce is when you buy it and how it was handled and stored through the distribution chain. But there are some things you can do.

Container Management

Produce should fill the container it's stored in. As you use or consume the produce, transfer what's left to a smaller container (see page 44 for more on this). This keeps the produce exposed to as little air as possible. This principle applies to raw and cooked produce alike.

You want to start with a well-fitted container from day one and you want to end with a well-fitted container (of much less food) on day 7, 10, 14, or otherwise. This is your best possible assurance of continued freshness.

If you struggle with condensation and humidity in your fridge, you can set a paper napkin or paper towel on top of your produce before sealing the container lid to absorb excess moisture. (*Ecofriendly tip:* You can use reusable cotton makeup-remover pads or cut-up dish towels in place of paper napkins or paper towels.) I'll note when doing this is generally advantageous. If you notice water buildup on your food storage lids, wipe those down midweek.

Container Placement

I will sometimes give you very specific guidance on storing produce in a warmer area of your fridge. Typically, this means pulled to the front of your shelves on a lower level or in the butter keeper on the door.

Midweek Rehydration

There's a reason there are usually misters in the produce section of the supermarket—a huge part of keeping produce fresh is maintaining its water content. For some storage techniques, like tenting (see page 82), you should change the water midweek or every 3 to 4 days. If you're using natural-fiber produce storage bags, it's a good idea to spritz them with a fine mist of water midweek to help keep the produce inside adequately hydrated.

Food-Grade Waxing

All plants naturally have a unique waxy layer known as the cuticle, which is present on the leaves of the plant and on any fruit it produces. The cuticle is a barrier against water loss, chemical attack, mechanical injury, and microbial infection. After harvest and before packaging, produce is repeatedly washed, which removes this natural waxy coating. So produce processors will often apply a layer of food-grade wax to help increase shelf life, prevent moisture loss and mechanical damage, and improve appearance.

Though commonly referred to as "waxes," these can be any number of waxes, oils, and/or resins. Examples include carnauba wax, beeswax, shellac (an insect wax), and petroleum-based waxes. Sometimes other chemicals are added. Waxes and edible coatings must be approved by the FDA and are applied to both conventional and organic produce. (Organic produce must be coated with specified organic waxes.) Petroleum and shellac aren't substances we'd normally want to consume, but the FDA assures us that these coatings are perfectly edible, and they're used in tiny amounts.

Any fresh produce that has been waxed must be labeled as such, typically on the signage displayed where the produce is stocked. Common wording might be "Coated with food-grade vegetable-, petroleum-, beeswax-, or shellac-based wax or resin, to maintain freshness." If you're not sure, you can always ask an associate in the produce department at your local supermarket. Wax is most often applied to:

- Apples
- Bell peppers
- Cucumbers
- Eggplants
- Grapefruits
- Lemons
- Limes
- Oranges
- Parsnips
- Passion fruits
- Peaches
- Potatoes
- Pumpkins
- Rutabagas
- Squash
- Sweet potatoes
- Tomatoes
- Turnips
- Yucca

There's no need to worry about removing food-grade wax before eating coated fruits or vegetables. Just rinse your produce under running water as usual. (If you *are* concerned about the wax, however, you can soak your produce—I provide some guidance on this in the section to come.) For cucumbers and other firm produce with a tougher rind, the FDA recommends scrubbing with a vegetable brush while rinsing under running water. You should do this even if you intend to peel the produce, especially cantaloupe. This reduces the risk that contaminants on the surface get into the flesh as you cut through the skin or otherwise handle the produce.

It's also worth noting that local farmers often don't wax their produce—yet another reason to frequent your local farmers' market!

Ethylene Compatibility Chart

Ethylene-Producing Foods

- Apples
- Apricots
- Avocados
- Ripening bananas
- Cantaloupe
- Cherimoyas
- Figs
- Honeydew
- Kiwifruits
- Mamey sapote
- Mangoes
- Mangosteen
- Nectarines
- Papayas
- Passion fruits
- Peaches
- Pears
- Persimmons
- Plantains
- Plums
- Prunes
- Quince
- Tomatoes

Ethylene-Sensitive Foods

- Unripe bananas
- Belgian endive
- Broccoli
- Brussels sprouts
- Cabbage
- Carrots
- Cauliflower
- Chard
- Cucumbers
- Eggplant
- Green beans
- Leafy greens
- Lettuce
- Okra
- Parsley
- Peas
- Peppers
- Spinach
- Squash
- Sweet potatoes
- Watercress
- Watermelon

General Ethylene Observations

In researching this book, I realized that nearly all of the available food science data relates particularly to industrial practices. This is especially true when it comes to ethylene. Ethylene interactions will not be as pronounced in your home fridge as they would be in a large cold-storage room. I've included this quick-check compatibility chart for your reference, but I don't want it to overwhelm or scare you. Here are the simple combination rules I have personally observed:

- **High-ethylene-producing fruit can still store well with other fruits.** For example: I store apples, citrus, plums, and pears all together in my crisper drawers without problems. I think this is because I store these fruits in my fridge once I get them from the store, without leaving them out on the counter to ripen first (which would increase respiration and ethylene production).
- **Ethylene-related problems in the home fridge are more likely when a fruit and veggie don't mix well together.** For example: broccoli stored next to ripe apples or pears in a crisper drawer.
- **Produce bags mitigate ethylene interactions.** If you are following the Fresh Fridge goal (see page 12) and plan to house most of your produce in your crisper drawers, just make sure you keep everything in individual plastic produce bags and you shouldn't have any issues.

Apples

Seasonality: Apple harvests in the US last from early August to early November. But we have access to apples year-round thanks to their long commercial cold storage life (3 to 6 months), plus imports.

Shopping: Because the majority of an apple's nutrients are found in its skin, it's a good idea to buy organic if your budget allows. Look for smooth, firm apples with vibrant coloration for their variety.

Prep and Storage

Washing: Commercial apples are coated with food-grade wax (see page 85). I like to fill a large bowl with hot water, add the apples we are going to eat for the week, and soak for at least 30 minutes, then rinse and dry them well. (You can add 1 tablespoon lemon juice or apple cider vinegar to the water if you wish to help remove more of the wax.)

Ethylene: Apples are very high ethylene producers (except for the Fuji and Granny Smith varieties). That's why you can use a ripe apple to help ripen other fruits. Just place 5 to 7 pieces of fruit you'd like to ripen in a bowl or bag with a ripe apple. Apples also have high ethylene sensitivity, but this is mostly a concern during long-term cold-chain storage, not at-home storage.

Optimal storage conditions: 32°F with 90 to 95% relative humidity

Room-temperature storage: Apples ripen 6 to 10 times faster at room temperature than if refrigerated. If you are eating them within 7 days, it's fine to keep them at room temp.

Whole: At room temperature (with favorable ambient conditions) for 1 to 2 weeks, or up to a month in the crisper drawer, loose (this is my preferred storage method, because my family likes apples chilled). Do not store apples in the same drawer as ethylene-sensitive produce, especially vegetables (see the chart on page 86). I've found loose unwashed apples store well in crisper drawers with both citrus and plums.

Sliced or shredded, with lemon juice added: 2 days in a glass food storage container

Artichokes

Seasonality: In the US, artichokes are predominantly grown in California, and their season lasts from March to June. A smaller crop is grown in October.

Shopping: Look for tightly closed heads. The leaves should be compact and the head should be firm.

Prep and Storage

Washing: Because I always eat my fresh artichokes steamed, I don't do anything special other than washing the artichokes just before I'm about to prepare them.

Ethylene: Artichokes have very low ethylene production and low ethylene sensitivity.

Optimal storage conditions: 32°F with 95% relative humidity

Whole: 5 to 7 days, wrapped with plastic or tented in a jar or container with a tablespoon of water at the bottom

Hearts, steamed: 3 to 5 days in a glass food storage container

Asparagus

Seasonality: In the US, asparagus is predominantly grown in California. Though it is available year-round, the US season lasts from February to June; April is peak asparagus season.

Shopping: Asparagus can dry out quickly. Look for spears that are green almost all the way through, with moist heads and stems. If a store or vendor is keeping their asparagus in chilled water or ice, that's a great sign.

Prep and Storage

Washing: Wash under cool water and snap off the woody bottom part of the stalks (the stalks will naturally break in the proper place). Dry with a dish towel before storing.

Ethylene: Asparagus has very low ethylene production but medium ethylene sensitivity. Due in part to its sensitivity, one rotting, bad, or aging spear can greatly affect the lifespan of the other vegetables stored with it.

Optimal storage conditions: 36°F with 95 to 100% relative humidity

Whole: 7 to 9 days standing upright in a glass jar filled with 2 inches of water, tenting with a plastic or silicone bag is optional but preferred especially in colder and drier areas of your fridge

Sliced, 2-inch-long pieces: 5 to 7 days in a glass food storage container

Steamed, whole: 5 to 7 days in a glass food storage container

QUICK MICROWAVE-STEAMED ASPARAGUS: Place washed, trimmed asparagus between two microwave-safe plates and microwave for 1 minute for crunchy spears or 90 seconds for tender stalks.

Avocados

Seasonality: Available year-round, Hass avocados are in season from March to September in the US. Florida avocados are available from summer through the winter months.

Types: There are two main types of avocados sold in the US: Hass avocados are smaller, with textured dark-green skin, and are commonly grown in Mexico and California. West Indies varieties (Pollock, Doni, Lula, and Bernecker) are larger, with smooth, shiny, bright green skin, and are predominantly grown in Florida.

Shopping: Avocados can ripen on or off the tree. Harder, lighter-colored avocados are less ripe (and will take 4 to 5 days to ripen). The navel of the avocado, where the small bit of stem remains, can help you assess ripeness, too: The looser the stem, the riper the avocado.

Prep and Storage

Ethylene: All types of avocados produce high amounts of ethylene and are also sensitive to ethylene.

Optimal storage conditions:

- Unripe mature Hass avocados: 37 to 45°F with 85 to 90% relative humidity

- Unripe mature Florida avocados: 55°F with 85 to 90% relative humidity

- Ripe avocados (any type): 36° to 40°F

Whole, unripe: Don't store unripe avocados in the fridge. Store at room temperature until ripe (until you can feel some give when you squeeze them), then transfer to the fridge to prolong shelf life.

Whole, ripe: averages 6 to 8 days in the fridge in a crisper drawer or storage bin

Halved, pit kept intact: 2 to 3 days in a glass container; the exposed flesh will darken

Halved, pit removed: 1 to 2 days stored in a silicone bag with the flesh pressed up against the side of the bag; exposed flesh will darken

Sliced, sprinkled with lime or lemon juice: 1 to 2 days in a glass food storage container. The acid in the citrus juice minimizes darkening.

Bananas

Seasonality: Bananas are available year-round. Almost all bananas sold in the US are imported from Costa Rica, Ecuador, Colombia, Honduras, Panama, or Guatemala. They are harvested unripe and green because they have to travel so far to market. They are then treated with ethylene gas for 1 to 2 days, which causes them to ripen and their skin to turn yellow.

Shopping: You can usually find both green and yellow bananas at the grocery store. I like to get a variety of ripeness levels to use throughout the week.

Prep and Storage

Ethylene: Bananas are medium ethylene producers and have a high sensitivity to ethylene. To ripen bananas quickly, place them in a paper bag. If you have a ripe apple, you can add it to the bag to increase the ethylene.

Optimal storage conditions: 55° to 59°F with 90 to 95% relative humidity

Whole: Room temperature storage is recommended. In warmer climates or seasons, bananas will ripen faster. You can store whole bananas in your refrigerator in these situations. The peels will turn black, but the fruit inside is still good to eat and will last longer overall. A helpful tip: Separate your bananas from the bunch, and store the loose bananas in a bowl or on a plate; this will help you avoid inadvertently tearing the peels later, which would cause them to ripen faster.

Frozen: Slice the bananas (or tear them in half) and arrange them on a tray or in a large gallon-size plastic bag. Freeze overnight, then transfer to an airtight plastic freezer container and store in the freezer at 0°F for 2 to 3 months. This is an especially good way to make use of very ripe/speckled bananas.

Bean Sprouts

Seasonality: Sprouts are available year-round, as beans are sprouted without soil or sunlight.

Shopping: Mung bean sprouts are commonly found in the refrigerated section of the produce department. They are small yellow-green beans with long white tails. Soy, lentil, and other types of bean sprouts aren't available in most supermarkets, but you can sprout your own at home.

Prep and Storage

Washing: Rinse with cool water before eating.

Ethylene: Technically, the plant is still in the growing stage, so respiration and ethylene production are not taking place.

Optimal storage conditions: Beans are sprouted at room temperature and then transferred to the fridge once their tails reach ½ inch long.

Mung bean sprouts, store-bought: 7 to 9 days in a glass jar filled with water plus 1 teaspoon lemon juice (or a few slices of lemon will work, too) or white vinegar; 5 days loosely stored in a dry glass container; 3 to 5 days rinsed and placed in a plastic storage bag with a paper towel

Lentil or soy sprouts, home-sprouted: 3 to 5 days in a glass container with a paper towel or washcloth at the bottom to soak up extra moisture. It's always wise to err on the side of caution with homegrown sprouts and eat them as quickly as ossible.

Beets

Seasonality: Red beets are usually available at supermarkets year-round. The US season typically lasts from November through the late winter months, including March and April.

Shopping: Fresh beets are sold in bunches with their greens attached or loose (also known as "topped") with the greens trimmed. Bunched beets are typically harvested earlier so the greens are fresher and in better condition. Loose beets are usually harvested later in their life cycle, since the root is the only thing that will be harvested. Look for firm roots and bright green leaves. Mud residue is typical for beets and doesn't mean they aren't safe or fresh. Smaller beets have tender skin that doesn't need to be peeled before eating.

Prep and Storage

Washing: I only wash beets when I'm ready to prepare them. Because beets are the plant's roots, they usually have a lot of mud and dirt debris that needs to be washed off. Fill your sink with cool water, add the beets, and move them around with your hand to release dirt, then let soak for at least 30 minutes. Rinse thoroughly with cool water, then dry with a dish towel before storing or using.

Ethylene: Beets are very low ethylene producers and have low ethylene sensitivity—this means they play very well with other produce.

Optimal storage conditions: 32°F with 98 to 100% relative humidity

Whole (unwashed): Up to a month (often much longer, in my experience). If you're looking to store your beets for a long time before using them, trim off and reserve the beet greens, place the beets in a plastic produce bag or zip-top plastic bag, and store in the crisper drawer.

Beet greens (unwashed): 9 to 12 days placing the greens upright in a glass jar with 2 inches of water at the bottom and tented loosely with a plastic bag, or for 5 to 7 days when you wash the greens, dry them completely, slice, and store in a glass food storage container.

Beet stems (washed): 9 to 12 days when left in long pieces and placed in a plastic zip-top bag or silicone bag. 5 to 7 days when diced and stored in a glass food container or jar. Similar to celery, there will be some fraying and drying on the cut ends. You can add water to the jar to combat this; the pigment from the stems will color the water, but they will still be fresh to eat.

Whole (washed): I only recommend prewashing whole beets if you intend to eat, cook, or pickle them within 7 days. Store washed whole beets (without their greens) in a plastic produce bag or zip-top plastic bag in the crisper drawer or in a large glass food storage container in the fridge for 5 to 7 days.

Shredded (raw): 4 to 6 days in a glass food storage container.

Shredded (roasted): 7 to 9 days in a glass food storage container or jar. Adding vinegar or lemon juice can extend shelf life for a couple more days.

Steamed (chopped): 5 to 7 days in a glass jar, or 7 to 9 days in a jar filled with water or enough steaming liquid (plus water as needed) to cover

Roasted (chopped): 7 to 9 days in a glass food storage container (see recipe, page 252)

Pickled: 2 to 3 weeks (see recipe, page 202)

Bell Peppers

Seasonality: Bell peppers are available year-round in US supermarkets; most are imported from Mexico and increasingly from Canadian greenhouses. Domestic bell pepper peak season runs from July to September.

Shopping: Because my family eats bell peppers raw and frequently, we always try to buy organic. Look for peppers that are firm and well colored—the deeper the color, the better. Avoid wrinkled or bruised peppers.

Prep and Storage

Washing: I only wash bell peppers when I'm getting ready to cut and store them for the week. I wash organic bell peppers under cool running water. Conventional bell peppers may have a petroleum-based wax coating applied (see page 85). If that's the case, you can soak the peppers in water mixed with 1 tablespoon lemon juice or apple cider vinegar to help remove the wax.

Ethylene: Bell peppers are low ethylene producers and have low ethylene sensitivity.

Optimal storage conditions: 45° to 50°F with 95 to 98% relative humidity

Whole (unwashed): 5 to 7 days loose, or 10 to 14 days in a plastic bag, in the crisper drawer. The best plastic storage bags for bell peppers are the shiny plastic type with holes, in which packaged bell peppers are often sold. Next best is a gallon-size zip-top plastic bag with about an inch of the top left open. They also store well in cotton or linen produce bags in the crisper drawer.

Sliced (1 inch thick): 7 to 9 days, laid flat in a glass food storage container or stored upright in a glass jar

Thinly sliced (¾ inch thick or less): 5 to 7 days stored upright in a glass jar or laid flat in a glass food storage container

Diced: 3 to 5 days in a glass jar, longer if you don't open and close the jar frequently

Berries

Seasonality: Fresh berries—strawberries, blackberries, blueberries, raspberries, and cranberries—are available at US supermarkets almost year-round (whether they taste great year-round is another issue), as imports from South America typically fill shelves when domestic berry seasons end. US blueberry season runs from April to late September. Strawberry season is highly dependent on where you live in the country but can run from January through November in some areas. Peak blackberry season is short, lasting only from July to August. Raspberries are in season from July to October (depending on location), and cranberries from mid-September until around mid-November.

Shopping: I always try to buy organic berries, as the skin is prone to holding pesticide residue. Frozen conventional berries are also a good choice, because they are not sprayed with fungicides after harvest. When buying fresh, pick the most darkly pigmented berries you can find, and look out for any signs of rot or mold. Any mushy or moldy berries in a pack will leave the other berries prone to premature rot.

Prep and Storage

Washing: For maximum shelf life, it is best to wait to wash berries until just before you plan to eat them. (Strawberries are the exception to this general rule; I have stored sliced washed strawberries with good results.) When I'm ready to enjoy berries, I simply rinse them with cool running water.

Ethylene: All berries are low ethylene producers and have low ethylene sensitivity.

Optimal storage conditions: All berry types prefer 90 to 95% relative humidity.

- Blackberries, blueberries, and raspberries: 31° to 32°F

- Strawberries: 32°F

- Cranberries: 35° to 41°F

Whole (unwashed):

- **Strawberries, blackberries, and blueberries:** Up to 7 days in the original plastic package, away from the airflow vents (to keep them from drying out too quickly). In my experience, berries stored in the crisper drawers get moldy faster (cranberries are the exception; see below). Blueberries will keep for 7 to 9 days in a glass jar. Ecofriendly storage option: Store berries unwashed in a shallow bowl or dish to provide plenty of breathing room; they can be left uncovered or you can drape them with a cloth or fitted fabric bowl cover.

- **Raspberries:** Softer berries tend to spoil the fastest—I'm lucky to get 3 or 4 days from supermarket raspberries. (Raspberries from your farmers' market may last longer.)

- **Cranberries:** 2 to 3 weeks in their original packaging or, if bought at a farmers' market, in a plastic bag, stored in the crisper drawer

Strawberries, washed and cut: 7 to 9 days. Rinse the berries and trim off their green tops. Halve smaller berries or quarter larger ones, then arrange them in a glass food storage container with a tight-fitting lid. (You can line the bottom of the container with a paper napkin or paper towel first.) This is how I like to prep our strawberries for the week, but note that they will be a bit dried out on their cut surfaces starting around day 3 or 4. My family doesn't mind this texture difference, but you might.

Frozen, all berries: Berries go bad quickly and are expensive in the off season, so it's a good idea to freeze your own during the summer months when they are the most delicious and plentiful! Line a large tray or flat container with parchment paper. Rinse the berries with cool water and dry gently with a dish towel, then arrange them on the tray or in the container and freeze them overnight. The next day, transfer them to a plastic freezer container with a tight-fitting lid to minimize freezer burn. If freezer burn is a particular problem for you, portion the frozen berries into silicone or plastic storage bags and house the bags in the container.

Bok Choy

Seasonality: The US supply of bok choy (also known as pak choi or Chinese white cabbage) is typically grown in California, and its lengthy season runs from April to December. Baby bok choy (Shanghai bok choy is one variety) is simply harvested earlier than full-grown bok choy and is about half the size. Baby bok choy grows best in the cool, shorter days of fall and early spring, so that's when you'll see it hitting the farmers' market.

Shopping: It is sweeter and less bitter than mature bok choy. For both, look for heads that are tight with clean, intact outer leaves. For baby bok choy, the greener the leaves, the better.

Prep and Storage

Washing: Fill your sink or a large bowl with cool water, add the trimmed bok choy (cut the bottom 1 to 1½ inches off the stalks), and soak, gently agitating the heads from time to time to release any sand or grit from the leaves.

Ethylene: Bok choy has very low ethylene production, but it has high ethylene sensitivity. When placed next to ethylene-producing produce, the bok choy leaves can turn yellow and toughen.

Optimal storage conditions: 32°F with 95 to 100% relative humidity

Whole (unwashed): Up to 2 weeks in a plastic bag; up to 3 weeks in a glass food storage container

Sliced: 12 to 14 days in a glass food storage container, tightly packed, with very little space for air

Sautéed: 9 to 12 days in a glass food storage container

SIMPLE SAUTÉED BABY BOK CHOY: Wash 5 or 6 baby bok choy and cut off the bottom inch to separate the heads into individual leaves. In a large pan or Dutch oven, heat 1 tablespoon veggie broth over medium-high heat. Add the bok choy and cook, stirring frequently and adding a splash more broth if the pan gets dry, for 3 to 5 minutes, until the leaves just begin to wilt. Reduce the heat to low and cook for 5 minutes more. Sprinkle with garlic powder and stir in 1 teaspoon coconut aminos (optional; use more if you prefer a stronger taste).

Serve immediately, or let cool and store in a glass food storage container for 9 to 12 days.

TIP: Store unused or damaged bok choy stalks and leaves in a bag in your freezer to use in Asian Veggie Scrap Broth (page 315).

Broccoli

Seasonality: Broccoli is available year-round in US supermarkets. Known as a winter vegetable, its peak season runs from October to April.

Shopping: Look for tightly closed, dark-green buds that are tightly packed to the broccoli head. Avoid heads with buds that are opening and/or yellowing—this means the broccoli is aged, and the flavor and texture will not be ideal. You can quickly tell the freshness of a broccoli head by looking at the cut end of the stalk—if it's brown, it's on the older side.

Prep and Storage

Washing: I only wash broccoli when I'm ready to process it for the week. First, give the whole head a rinse under cool water. Cut the florets from the stalk and chop them, then rinse the chopped florets again. I do this double rinse because small bugs called cabbage aphids can commonly hang out in broccoli and other cruciferous veggies. If you happen to have a stalk with quite a few aphids, you can soak the florets in a large bowl of water with lemon juice or apple cider vinegar. Don't let the aphids get you down—broccoli is a nutritious, alive food, so it shouldn't be a surprise that the aphids are all about it.

Ethylene: Broccoli has very low ethylene production but high ethylene sensitivity. When placed next to ethylene-producing produce, the buds will start to open and become inedible.

Optimal storage conditions: 32°F with 95 to 100% relative humidity

Whole (unwashed): 10 to 12 days in a plastic produce bag in the crisper drawer or on the middle or lower shelf

Chopped (florets and/or stalks): 7 to 9 days in a glass food storage container or glass jars. The finer you chop the broccoli, the less time it will stay fresh; larger florets stay fresh longer. Broccoli stalks are just as nutritious as the florets, so there's no need to throw them away! I love chopping them into spears and eating with hummus or guac. (If you cut them into spears, store them in a glass jar filled with water to prevent them from drying out.)

Lightly steamed: 9 to 12 days in a glass food storage container

LIGHTLY STEAMED BROCCOLI: Chop fresh broccoli into florets and rinse well—do not dry. Place in a microwave-safe bowl and add no more than 1½ teaspoons water. Cover with another microwave-safe bowl or plate and microwave for 1 minute. If cooking more than 1 cup of florets, allow them to rest for 20 seconds, then microwave for 30 seconds more and test for doneness; the broccoli should be bright green and still crunchy. For a more tender result, microwave in additional 30-second intervals, testing after each until you reach the desired doneness. Serve, or let cool and store in the fridge in a glass food storage container for 9 to 12 days.

TIP: Store unused or damaged broccoli stalks and leaves in a bag in your freezer to use in Asian Veggie Scrap Broth (page 315).

Brussels Sprouts

Seasonality: Brussels sprouts are available year-round in US supermarkets. Commonly thought of as a fall vegetable, their peak season runs from September to mid-February.

Shopping: Brussels sprouts are typically much fresher when you buy them still on the stalk. Either way, look for compact, tight, firm buds with a uniform green color. Avoid yellowing leaves and splitting outer leaves (which indicate that the sprouts are overmature and likely more bitter). I've found that the sweetest-tasting Brussels sprouts are usually no more than 1 inch in diameter.

Prep and Storage

Washing: Because Brussels sprouts grow up away from the soil and their buds are tightly formed, you don't have to worry too much about dirt and debris. I typically trim the ends and rinse the outside of the sprouts with cool running water or let them soak in a large bowl of water for a bit, then gently pat dry with a dish towel before preparing or processing them.

Ethylene: Brussels sprouts have very low ethylene production but high ethylene sensitivity. When stored next to ethylene-producing produce, Brussels sprouts will overmature and turn bitter.

Optimal storage conditions: 32°F with 95 to 100% relative humidity

Whole (unwashed): While Brussels sprouts will keep for 10 to 12 days in the fridge, their taste is best when cooked or eaten raw within a week. If purchased on the stalk, leave intact, if possible, to preserve flavor and shelf life; store the whole stalk in a large plastic bag in the crisper drawer. Loose Brussels sprouts store very well in linen or cotton food storage bags in the crisper drawer—the natural fibers of the bags maintain optimal water content while absorbing any excess water that can cause the leaves to rot.

Halved: 7 to 9 days in a glass food storage container or glass jar, but to retain their inherent sweetness, it's best to cook or eat cut (halved or shaved) Brussels sprouts within 3 days.

Shaved: 5 to 7 days in a glass food storage container or glass jar

Steamed or roasted: 7 to 9 days in a glass food storage container with little air exposure

LIGHTLY STEAMED BRUSSELS SPROUTS: Use the same method outlined for steaming broccoli (see page 99).

SIMPLE NO-OIL ROASTED BRUSSELS SPROUTS: Preheat the oven to 375°F. Line a baking sheet with parchment paper. Halve enough Brussels sprouts to make about 3 cups. In a large bowl, combine the Brussels sprouts and ½ cup Tahini Yum Sauce (page 172) and toss well. Arrange in a single layer on the prepared baking sheet and roast for about 35 minutes, until fork-tender and just beginning to brown, rotating the pan once halfway through.

Cabbage

Seasonality: Cabbage (red, green, and napa) is available year-round in US supermarkets. Commonly thought of as a fall vegetable, its peak season runs from September to November. Much of the cabbage crop is harvested in the fall and then put into cold storage to make it available through spring.

Shopping: Look for firm, compact heads that are intensely colored. The outer leaves may be a bit beaten up, but that doesn't mean the cabbage is bad; those leaves will be removed anyway. You can also gauge freshness by flipping the head over and taking a look at the cut stem—if it's browning, the cabbage may be on the older side. But keep in mind that cabbage can be stored for months before reaching grocery store shelves. I'll put it this way: I've never encountered a "bad" cabbage.

Prep and Storage

Washing: Because cabbages are tightly formed, they don't collect much dirt or debris. Remove one or two layers of the outer leaves and then rinse under cool running water. For red cabbage, I like to quarter the head through the stalk end. From there, I can cut the cabbage into thick or thin slices or separate the individual leaves to make cabbage "cups." For napa cabbage, I cut the cabbage in half through the stalk end and then thinly slice.

Ethylene: Cabbage has very low ethylene production but high sensitivity; napa cabbage has medium sensitivity.

Optimal storage conditions: 32°F with 98 to 100% relative humidity for red and green cabbage, 95 to 100% relative humidity for napa cabbage

Whole (unwashed): 1 month, uncovered, in the crisper drawer. You can extend this to 1½ to 2 months if you wrap the head in plastic wrap or house it in a large plastic bag with air removed.

Halved or quartered: 2 to 3 weeks in a plastic, cotton, or linen bag in the crisper drawer

Thick slices or large dice: 14 to 16 days in a glass food storage container or glass jar— I consistently get up to 3 weeks.

Thinly sliced: 8 to 10 days in a glass food storage container with little air exposure

Lightly steamed: 7 to 9 days in a glass food storage container

Carrots

Seasonality: Carrots are available year-round in US supermarkets, and their peak season runs from the summer to the fall.

Shopping: You'll find carrots loose (tops removed, bagged) or bunched (with the greens intact). No matter which type you're shopping for, look for firm carrots with even, bright color. Watch out for carrots that are limp (this means they have lost moisture) or that have a black ring around the carrot top where the greens emerge from the root—that's a sign they aren't as fresh. Smaller carrots are usually more tender and larger carrots are sweeter and crunchier. If you're buying bunched carrots, look for carrot greens with unbroken stems and pert, lively leaves (wilted carrot greens signify that the carrots weren't stored with enough humidity).

Prep and Storage

Washing: Because carrots are root vegetables and grown in the ground, you really want to give them a thorough wash. I typically fill my sink or a large bowl with warm water and scrub the carrots with a brush. When I'm ready to use the greens, I give them a rinse under cool running water.

Ethylene: Carrots have very low ethylene production but high ethylene sensitivity.

Optimal storage conditions: 32°F with 98 to 100% relative humidity

Whole (unwashed): 3 weeks in a plastic storage bag in the crisper drawer, or 2 weeks in cotton or linen produce bags in the crisper drawer. If you buy bunched carrots, cut off the greens before storing the carrots. The greens will spoil much more quickly than the roots and will contribute to water loss in the root if they're kept attached. Store the unwashed greens separately in a plastic, cotton, or linen bag in the crisper drawer for 3 to 5 days, or freeze in an airtight freezer container or plastic bag (wash them first) for 4 to 6 weeks.

Cut into sticks: 10 to 12 days (I've even gotten up to 2 weeks) stored in a glass jar filled with water; or 7 to 9 days without the water (they may dry out slightly toward the end of the week).

Diced or sliced: 7 to 9 days in a glass food storage container or glass jar. You can fill the container with water if you'd like to eke out a few more days of storage before cooking.

Shredded: 5 to 7 days in a glass food storage container or glass jar with little air exposure

Lightly steamed: 7 to 9 days in a glass food storage container

Greens, blanched: 5 to 7 days in a glass food storage container or glass jar with little air exposure

QUICK CARROT GREENS PESTO: Remove the greens from 1 bunch of carrots and rinse well; dry with a dish towel. Place in a food processor and add 1 garlic clove (pressed or chopped); ½ cup pine nuts, cashews, walnuts, or hulled pumpkin seeds; 3 tablespoons lemon juice; 1 cup packed baby spinach; and salt and ground black pepper to taste. Process for 5 seconds, then scrape down the sides with a spatula. Add up to 2 tablespoons olive oil, if desired, and pulse until a smooth paste is formed. You can also add 1 teaspoon lemon zest and up to ¼ cup fresh mint, if desired. Store in the fridge in a glass jar for up to 5 days. I love serving this in the spring with roasted carrots and radishes.

Cauliflower

Seasonality: Cauliflower is available year-round in US supermarkets; in many farmers' markets, you can find it even in traditionally out-of-season months. Peak season runs from September to November. In the US, 90% of all cauliflower is grown in California, with the rest grown in Arizona and New York. (Romanesco can be stored using these same methods as well.)

Shopping: Look for a firm, compact head that's at least 6 inches wide, with uniformly colored curds (those are the tops of the florets). The head should be surrounded by green leaves—look for brightly colored leaves that are tight against the cauliflower head. Overmature heads will have loose or protruding floral parts that create a fuzziness on the top of the head. Patches of pale brown discoloration are a common defect on cauliflower heads, but aren't an indication that the veggie isn't good quality. The brown spots are oxidation that happens during storage after harvest—the longer the cauliflower is stored, the more likely it is to have these spots. Just cut them off the surface of the cauliflower, and you're good to go. You only really need to worry if the spots turn dark and get slimy—then it's time to ditch the cauliflower.

Prep and Storage

Washing: Rinse the head under cool running water.

Ethylene: Cauliflower have very low ethylene production, but they have high ethylene sensitivity.

Optimal storage conditions: 32°F with 95 to 98% relative humidity

Whole (unwashed): 21 days in a plastic storage bag or the original perforated plastic wrapping in the crisper drawer (note that when stored this long, there will be some oxidative browning on the surface), or 10 to 14 days in a cotton or linen produce bag in the crisper drawer

Florets: 10 to 12 days (I've even gotten up to 2 weeks) in a glass food storage container or glass jar. Cut off any browning spots, then cut the head in half and remove the florets from the stalk.

TIP: Save the stalks to make riced cauliflower. Pulse the washed and dried stalks in a food processor.

Riced or diced: 5 to 7 days in a glass food storage container or glass jar, tightly packed, with little air exposure

Lightly steamed (florets): 7 to 9 days in a glass food storage container

Steamed (riced): 5 to 7 days in a glass food storage container

Celery

Seasonality: Celery is grown year-round in the US, with the vast majority grown in California and some in Michigan. It's a difficult veggie to grow, as it takes a long time to reach maturity and requires lots of water and cooler temperatures.

Shopping: I've found the greenest celery tends to be the tastiest celery. When you're buying a bunch, be on the lookout for any brown spots or yellowing on the outer leaves, as well as shriveling at the cut tops or cracking along the length of the stalks— this means the celery's a bit older.

Prep and Storage

Washing: I only wash my celery when I'm ready to process it. I like to fill my kitchen sink with cool water and let the celery soak for a bit, then give it a rinse under cool water.

Ethylene: Celery has very low ethylene production and medium ethylene sensitivity.

Optimal storage conditions: 32°F with 98 to 100% relative humidity

Whole (unwashed): 3 weeks in a plastic storage bag (it's a great idea to poke a few holes in the bag for breathing) or 2 weeks in cotton or linen produce bags in the crisper drawer (you need to lightly spray these bags with water every 4 days for long-term storage)

Cut into sticks: 7 to 9 days in a glass food storage container or glass jar with 1 to 2 inches of water at the bottom, or 10 to 12 days fully submerged in water (the cut ends may start to fray with longer storage)

Sliced or diced: 5 to 7 days in a glass food storage container or glass jar, tightly packed, with little air exposure. Discoloration is common toward the end of shelf life. Diced or sliced celery can also be stored in a glass food storage container, fully or partially submerged in water, for 6 to 9 days to ensure crispness (fraying is common). Diced celery can also be frozen like berries (see page 96) and can be cooked from frozen in sautés and soups. It keeps in the freezer for up to 2 months.

TIP: I sometimes use beet green stems or chard stems as a substitute for celery.

Cherries

Seasonality: Sweet cherries are available from May to August. Sour cherries have a shorter season, lasting for a few weeks in June, or in July or August for cooler areas of the country.

Shopping: Look for plump cherries, brightly colored for their variety, with as many green stems attached as possible.

Prep and Storage

Washing: Don't wash cherries until you're ready to eat them. I usually soak them for 10 minutes in cool water before we eat them.

Ethylene: Cherries have very low ethylene production and low ethylene sensitivity. You can store them anywhere in your fridge around other types of produce without worrying about adverse effects.

Optimal storage conditions: 30° to 32°F with 90 to 95% relative humidity

Whole, stems intact (unwashed): 10 to 14 days in a plastic, cotton, or linen bag in the fridge. I often keep cherries in an open dish or jar because my family eats them so quickly.

Whole (washed), unpitted: 3 to 5 days in a glass food storage container or glass jar.

Pitted: 2 to 3 days in a glass food storage container or glass jar, tightly packed, with little air exposure

Frozen (pitted): Up to 3 months in an airtight container

- **Pitting Techniques**: We're a spit-out-the-pit type of family, but I sometimes pit the cherries before storage as a special treat for the kids or if I'm going to freeze them. My favorite technique is inserting a straw at the top of the cherry and pushing it straight through. You can also insert the end of a paperclip into the top and hook the pit up and out.

Cilantro

Seasonality: Cilantro is available in the US all year long. The majority of the commercial cilantro crop is grown in California.

Shopping: Look for cilantro bunches that are brightly and deeply green. Fragrant leaves are a great indicator of freshness. Avoid bunches with wilted, yellowing, or black leaves.

Prep and Storage

Washing: Don't wash cilantro until you're ready to use it. I usually run it under cool water just before use.

Ethylene: Cilantro has very low ethylene production but high ethylene sensitivity. Avoid storing it next to high-ethylene-producing produce like apples or pears.

Optimal storage conditions: 32° to 34°F with 95 to 100% relative humidity

Whole (unwashed): Cilantro happens to be the number one herb I'm asked about storing in the fridge, because it's so darn fussy! I like to think of a bunch of fresh cilantro as a bouquet of delicate flowers. Remove any leaves from the bottom of the bunch, then stand it upright in a glass jar filled halfway with water and tent it with a plastic bag; stored this way, it will keep for 9 to 14 days. The tenting technique gives cilantro all its favorite things: humidity and space for its leaves to breathe. When you need to use some, simply tear a handful or two of leaves off the bunch (leaving the stems in the jar). After 5 or 6 days, change the water in the jar and remove any soggy leaves from the stem area. I also like to wipe down any condensation on the plastic bag when I change the water. If you buy cilantro in a small plastic clamshell, leave it in the original packaging and store it in the crisper drawer or butter keeper, where it will keep for 5 to 7 days.

Cut: 2 to 3 days in a glass food storage container or glass jar, tightly packed, with little air exposure

Citrus

Seasonality: Common citrus fruits like oranges, lemons, and limes are available in the US year-round, with gaps in domestic crops supplemented with fruits from South America. As a general rule, November through early spring is peak season for citrus. More specialty types of citrus have more distinct seasonality. For example, Sumo Citrus and navel orange season lasts from January to April, and Valencia oranges are in season in June and July.

Shopping: Unlike most fruits, a citrus fruit's skin color isn't necessarily an indicator of sweetness. Some of the sweetest and most flavorful oranges I've ever enjoyed had less-than-stellar skin color. Instead of coloration, look for firm fruit that gives just a little when squeezed. Watch out for mold (often found at the bottom of bagged oranges) and soft spots, as these will lead to premature spoilage. If you're going to zest the skin, make sure to purchase organic citrus.

Prep and Storage

Washing: If you don't plan to use the skin, you can skip washing citrus fruits. Otherwise, when you're ready to zest the citrus, or if you are cutting it with the skin on, soak it in warm water for 10 minutes and lightly scrub the skin with a brush, if desired, then dry. With my homegrown lemons, I like to soak them in cool water in the sink for 20 to 30 minutes then dry them completely in order to cool them down before long-term storage in the fridge.

Ethylene: Citrus has very low ethylene production, except for the sour Seville orange, which produces a bit more. All citrus varieties have medium ethylene sensitivity, so it's a good idea to keep them separate from high ethylene producers. One exception to this is apples. For years I have stored loose, unwashed citrus and apples together in the crisper drawer and it has not affected long-term storage duration.

Optimal storage conditions:

- **Grapefruit:** 50° to 59°F with 85 to 90% relative humidity

- **Lemons:** 50° to 55°F with 85 to 90% relative humidity

- **Limes:** 48° to 50°F with 85 to 90% relative humidity

- **Oranges (FL):** 32° to 36°F with 85 to 90% relative humidity

- **Oranges (CA, AZ):** 38° to 48°F with 85 to 90% relative humidity

- **Blood oranges:** 40° to 44°F with 90 to 95% relative humidity

- **Tangerines and mandarins:** 40° to 45°F with 90 to 95% relative humidity

Whole: 2 to 3 weeks in the crisper drawer, loose. Many sources recommend storing citrus on your kitchen counter at room temperature. But as you can see from the temperatures above, the fridge is actually a better choice. For homegrown citrus I've noticed extra shelf life when you keep ¼ to ½ inch stem intact.

Peeled mandarin segments: 7 to 9 days in a glass food storage container with a tight-fitting lid, tightly packed, with little air exposure. I like to peel mandarins for the week to make lunches and snacks easier.

Quartered oranges (skin on): 3 to 5 days in a glass food storage container with a tight-fitting lid, tightly packed, with little air exposure

Lemon or lime juice: 3 to 6 months in a glass jar with very little air exposure, placed at the back of your fridge closest to the airflow source. Replace the jar lid with a clean one every 2 months to prevent mold from forming on the lid. I've had hand-squeezed lemon juice keep for 9 months using this method. If that seems too extreme to you, know that your fresh-squeezed lime or lemon juice will be good for at least 2 weeks. Lemon or lime juice can also be frozen in a glass jar or into cubes for 9 to 12 months.

Collard Greens

Seasonality: Collard greens are available year-round in the US, with their peak lasting from January to April.

Shopping: If you're planning on cooking your collard greens, they are tastiest when harvested young (less than 10 inches long) and have a dark green leaf color. If you're using collard greens for wraps, look for the longest and widest leaves possible. Avoid wilting, cracked, torn, brown, or yellowing leaves.

Prep and Storage

Washing: Collard greens can sometimes be sandy. When I'm cooking or steaming a bunch, I'll soak the leaves in cool water in the sink for 10 minutes, then rinse with cool water and quickly pat them dry with a dish towel. When I'm just preparing one or two leaves, I'll rinse them with cool water, then scrub lightly with a dish towel.

Ethylene: Collard greens have very low ethylene production but high ethylene sensitivity.

Optimal storage conditions: 32°F with 95 to 100% relative humidity

Whole (unwashed): 9 to 12 days in a plastic produce bag or large zip-top bag (leaves may begin to yellow toward the end of this time), or 5 to 7 days in a linen bag (it's a good idea to spritz the bag with water midway through the week with this method)

Sliced or chopped: 3 to 5 days in a glass food storage container or glass jar, loosely packed, with little air exposure

Steamed: 7 to 9 days in a glass food storage container or glass jar, tightly packed, with little air exposure

QUICK MICROWAVE-STEAMED COLLARD GREENS: Rinse 4 or 5 large collard green leaves; do not dry them (that moisture will be used while steaming). Remove and discard the center stems and cut the leaves into ribbons or coarsely chop. Place in a microwave-safe bowl and add no more than 1½ teaspoons water. Cover with another microwave-safe bowl of the same size or a plate and heat for 1 minute. Allow to rest for 20 seconds, then heat on high for another 30 seconds. Test for doneness. The collards should be bright green and just soft, not mushy or soggy.

Corn

Seasonality: Sweet corn hits its peak between July and September. Depending on the temperatures in a particular year, the rest of the corn crop is harvested between September and November.

Shopping: Buying organic corn is best to avoid exposure to harmful chemicals from pesticides. When determining freshness, the easiest way would be to open the husk and take a peek at the kernels inside—but unfortunately, that's not good form at the supermarket! Instead, look for bright green, sometimes damp husks that stick tightly to the ear. I also look at the stringy tassels. They should be brown (not black) and sticky to the touch—a surefire way to know the corn is fresh!

Prep and Storage

Washing: Not necessary when you buy corn with the husk intact. If you buy shucked corn, it's not a bad idea to run it under cool water before preparing it.

Ethylene: Sweet corn has very low ethylene production and low ethylene sensitivity.

Optimal storage conditions: 32°F with 95 to 98% relative humidity

Whole, with husk: 7 to 9 days in the crisper drawer, loose. However, for the best flavor, eat or cook the corn quickly (within 3 days). As the corn respirates, the sugars will be converted to starch (and the corn will taste less sweet).

Whole, shucked: 3 to 5 days in a plastic bag or glass food storage container, if you shucked the ears yourself. Keep store-bought pre-shucked corn in its original packaging and eat it sooner—within 2 to 3 days.

Steamed or boiled (on the cob): 3 to 5 days in a glass food storage container placed toward the back of the fridge near an airflow source

Steamed, boiled or thawed from frozen (kernels): 5 to 7 days in a glass food storage container, tightly packed, with little air exposure

TIP: When sweet corn is at its peak, you can slice the raw kernels off the cob and store in a glass food container or jar for up to 7 days. Corn kernels can also be frozen from fresh after shucked (just like berries and celery; see page 96) and keep well in the freezer for 2 to 3 months.

Cucumber

Seasonality: Cucumbers are available year-round in the US, with their peak season running from May to August. Most of the cucumbers grown in the US come from Florida and Michigan.

Types: There are two major categories of cucumber: slicing and pickling. Slicing cucumbers are longer and have thicker skin to help them store longer; they are typically eaten raw. Pickling cucumbers are shorter, with thinner skin that allows them to absorb the flavor of the pickling brine.

Shopping: I recommend buying organic, as conventional cucumbers may have high levels of pesticide residues. Look for uniformly green cucumbers that don't have wrinkled tips or soft spots on the body.

Prep and Storage

Washing: Cucumbers are typically waxed (see page 85) or, in the case of English cucumbers, enclosed in a tight plastic sheath to help prolong shelf life and reduce moisture loss (cucumbers have the highest water content of any vegetable). To remove the wax (if desired), soak the cucumbers in a bowl of tepid water with 1 tablespoon distilled white vinegar for at least 15 minutes, then brush the skin thoroughly with a washcloth or vegetable brush to help remove the waxy residue. If you get cucumbers at a farmers' market, they are typically unwaxed.

Ethylene: Cucumbers have low ethylene production but high ethylene sensitivity.

Optimal storage conditions:

- Slicing cucumbers: 50° to 54°F with 85 to 90% relative humidity

- Pickling cucumbers: 40°F with 95 to 100% relative humidity

Whole (unwashed): 7 to 9 days in the original plastic or in a plastic, cotton, or linen bag in the crisper drawer

Large slices (½ inch thick): 5 to 7 days stacked in a glass food storage container with a tight-fitting lid. This is my preferred method of storing English cucumbers for the week. I also like to peel some of the skin to create a striped pattern (just for fun). The edges of the slices will dry out slightly over the week, but the interior will still be moist. If the dryness bothers you, take a wet paper towel or napkin, wring out excess moisture, and lay it in the bottom of the container before stacking the slices inside.

Diced: 4 to 6 days in a glass food storage container or glass jar, tightly packed

Thinly sliced, shredded, or spiralized: 3 to 5 days in a glass food storage container or glass jar. To double the shelf life with these cuts, you can add distilled white vinegar and toss well (a tip my mother-in-law taught me); I store them this way on weeks that I want to stretch my preps to 10 to 12 days. I enjoy adding these quasi-pickled cucumbers to my salads.

Eggplant

Seasonality: Eggplant is available year-round in the US, with peak season running from July to October. Eggplant is considered a summer crop, but in warmer regions of the country, it can be harvested in the fall and spring, too.

Shopping: The most common eggplant variety sold in the US is called Black Beauty—this type has purple-black skin with an oval or teardrop shape. Asian eggplant has a brighter purple skin and a long, slender shape. Farmers' markets may have other varieties, including smaller sizes. No matter the variety, look for eggplants that feel heavy for their size, with glossy, firm skin. Watch out for soft spots, brown discoloration, or wrinkling skin. Eggplants are typically waxed, so I prefer to buy organic or unwaxed eggplants at the farmers' market (ask your vendor).

Prep and Storage

Washing: If desired, soak eggplant in the sink or in a large bowl in warm water to loosen the wax. Then rinse them with warm water and buff off the waxy residue with a washcloth.

Ethylene: Eggplant has low ethylene production and medium ethylene sensitivity.

Optimal storage conditions: 50° to 54°F with 90 to 95% relative humidity

Whole (unwashed): 6 to 8 days in a plastic produce bag or 5 to 7 days in a cotton or linen produce bag. To avoid chilling injuries, store eggplant in the warmest part of your fridge, such as toward the front of a crisper drawer (away from an airflow source) or in the lower door storage area. Chilling injuries occur at temperatures lower than 45°F and take about 5 days to develop; they will most likely result in the browning of the inner seeds (which negatively affects the eggplant's flavor and texture). If your climate and ambient temperature allow (with daytime temperatures within 15°F of the optimal storage temperature above), you can store eggplant on your counter for up to 2 days.

Large dice: 2 to 4 days in a glass food storage container with very little air exposure. Do not place in the coldest parts of your fridge. I typically prep and store diced eggplant 1 or 2 days before cooking it.

Sliced ("lasagna noodles" and cooked [see below]): 2 to 4 days before preparing a finished dish, in a plastic bag or glass food storage container. Release any air in the bag or pack snugly with little air in the container.

HOW TO MAKE EGGPLANT LASAGNA "NOODLES": Select 2 large, wide eggplants; wash and dry. Preheat the oven to 375°F. Line a baking sheet with parchment paper or a silicone baking mat. Cut the top and bottom off an eggplant and stand it on one end on a cutting board. Slice it lengthwise into ¼-inch-thick slices (aim for 6 to 8 slices). Place the slices in a single layer on the prepared baking sheet and repeat with the second eggplant (if you need more room, line a second baking sheet). Bake for 20 minutes, until softened and lightly browned. Use to make lasagna with your favorite fillings and marinara sauce. Reserve the trimmings for roasting.

Roasted, chopped: 7 to 9 days in a glass food storage container or glass jar

Garlic

Seasonality: Garlic is available year-round in the US, with its peak season in summer. Most domestic garlic is grown in California, though some is grown in Oregon, Nevada, Washington, and New York. The US is the world's largest importer of garlic, so you may also see garlic from China, Argentina, and Mexico at your supermarket.

Shopping: Look for plump, firm, heavy heads of garlic with smooth, unbroken skin. The skin should be well "cured," meaning the neck and outer layers of skin are dry. Look out for heads with damp or soft spots or that feel light and dried out.

Prep and Storage

Ethylene: Garlic has very low ethylene production and low ethylene sensitivity.

Optimal storage conditions: 30° to 32°F with 65 to 70% relative humidity

Whole head: 2 to 3 weeks in a dark, cool, dry place. Keep away from light to prevent sprouting. I store heads of garlic in wooden storage bins that are lidded but not airtight, which allows for airflow. If your indoor climate is unusually humid or hot, you're best off buying new garlic weekly and prepping it to keep in the fridge as described below. Storing whole garlic heads in the fridge mimics the plant's early growing conditions (garlic is planted in the fall before the first early frosts) and will cause sprouting.

Whole cloves, peeled: 7 to 9 days in a small glass food storage container or glass jar. If you don't plan to use the garlic right away, keep it in a warmer part of your fridge—door storage is a good option.

PEELING GARLIC: Undoubtedly, peeling is the most tedious part of using fresh garlic, but I've learned a few methods that have helped make it less so. My mother-in-law takes skin-on cloves and soaks them in water for a day; after draining, the skins come off easily and with less of a crispy mess. Another method is to put the cloves in a glass jar, close the lid, and shake vigorously; most of the skins will come off and you can easily collect the peeled cloves. When roasting, leave the skins on, then you just squeeze out the roasted garlic inside.

Minced or grated: 5 to 7 days in a small glass food storage container or glass jar. Once the cloves are cut, you want to keep them in a cooler area of the fridge. If you've found your fridge conditions generally only allow for shorter shelf life, you can add a bit of lemon juice to aid preservation.

Roasted: 7 to 9 days in glass food storage container or glass jar

ROASTED GARLIC: Preheat the oven to 350°F. Put unpeeled garlic cloves in a baking dish or spread them over a baking sheet lined with parchment paper or a silicone baking mat. Roast for 25 to 30 minutes; you'll smell their amazing aroma around the 20-minute mark. The skins will start to crack toward the end of the cooking time and should just be beginning to brown. Remove from the oven and allow to cool completely. You can easily remove the skins from the cloves, or simply squeeze the softened garlic out of the skins. Discard the skins, or save them in the freezer to use for broth!

TIP: Save garlic skins and scraps to use in Veggie Scrap Broth (page 312).

Ginger and Turmeric

Seasonality: Ginger is considered a winter crop, while turmeric is a fall crop. Typically, you can find both of these roots year-round in your supermarket's produce department.

Shopping: If buying loose roots, choose those with smooth, shiny skin; avoid pieces with wrinkly, cracked skin. If you can only find ginger or turmeric in small plastic clamshells, you won't have much opportunity to assess freshness. In this case, look for the "best by" date on the packaging, and don't buy any with mold or shriveled ends.

Prep and Storage

Special Note on Turmeric: I couldn't find reliable ethylene, temperature, or humidity data for turmeric root. However, because it is similar in structure to ginger, it's a safe assumption that the numbers are very similar.

Washing: For ginger, since the skin is usually peeled, I only give it a quick rinse (if you peel turmeric, too, do the same). I typically scrub turmeric, as I like to keep the skin on when I grate it (if you keep the skin on your ginger, scrub it as well).

Ethylene: Ginger has very low ethylene production and low ethylene sensitivity.

Optimal storage conditions: 55°F with 65% relative humidity

Whole: 14 to 18 days in a plastic clamshell, plastic bag, or glass food storage container. Store ginger and turmeric in a warmer part of your fridge; my favorite spot for them is the butter keeper on the door. Once you cut off a piece, the shelf life will decrease to 7 to 9 days. Fresh ginger keeps well in the freezer in an airtight container or freezer bag for up to 6 months. It's easy to peel and grate frozen; return any unused portion to the freezer. If slicing, thaw it at room temperature first.

Peeled and grated or minced: 5 to 7 days in a small glass food storage container or glass jar. Keep in a cooler part of your fridge. If you've found your fridge conditions generally only allow for shorter shelf life, you can always add a bit of lemon or lime juice to aid preservation.

Grains

Cooked whole grains are a weekly staple in my fridge. Whole grains have only their indigestible outer hull removed; the nutrient-rich bran and germ remain intact. Intact whole grains include barley, steel-cut and rolled oats, brown rice, wild rice, quinoa, cracked wheat, wheat berries, rye berries, amaranth, sorghum, and millet. Here are storage guidelines for some of the most common.

Prep and Storage

Cooked rice, hulled barley, oatmeal, and quinoa (cooked in water): 9 to 12 days in a glass food storage container or glass jar, packed, with as little air exposure as possible. As you eat the grains throughout the week, downsize the container. I also like to portion 1-cup servings into smaller containers instead of one large container. If you know you're going to be eating the grains later in the week, store them toward the back of the fridge closer to an airflow source so they'll stay colder. Cooked grains can also be frozen in a glass food storage container for 4 to 6 weeks. Thaw in the fridge overnight. Reheat thoroughly; any leftover previously frozen grains can be stored in the fridge and eaten within 2 days.

EASY NOURISH BOWLS: This is my favorite, no-fuss way to enjoy whole grains, and it's why I always have a batch of cooked grain in my fridge or freezer! Portion 1 to 1½ cups of your favorite cooked whole grain into an individual serving bowl; add a cooked green vegetable, a lightly steamed or roasted colorful vegetable (like carrot, beet, eggplant, bell pepper), and one of my Plant-Based Proteins (pages 270–279); and top with your favorite sauce or hummus.

Grapes

Seasonality: Grapes are available in US supermarkets through most of the year, but the season runs from May to October, with peak season in September. Fall grapes are particularly delicious because grapes love warm weather, and the fruit spends the summer hanging on the vine, resulting in high sugar content and complex flavors.

Shopping: Pay attention to the stem condition when selecting bunches of grapes. When freshly harvested, stems are bright green and full, but as the fruit ages, the stems start to thin, dry out, and turn brown. Look for bunches with healthy green (or as close to green as you can get) stems and no broken, shriveled, cracked, or leaky grapes.

Prep and Storage

Washing: You'd be surprised how much dust and sediment can be lurking in a bunch of grapes. I like to soak them in a large bowl with cool water for about 20 minutes.

Ethylene: Grapes have very low ethylene production and low ethylene sensitivity.

Optimal storage conditions: 31° to 32°F with 90 to 95% relative humidity

Whole bunches (unwashed): 10 to 12 days in a plastic, cotton, or linen bag in the crisper drawer, or 7 to 9 days with vines left intact in a shallow bowl uncovered in the fridge

Whole bunches (washed): 5 to 7 days, left whole or cut into smaller bunches with vines intact and placed in an uncovered bowl on a lower shelf in the fridge, or 7 to 9 days in a glass food storage container. You can place a napkin or paper towel at the bottom of the container to combat excess humidity or moisture in your fridge.

Stemmed whole grapes (washed): 3 to 5 days in a glass food storage container or glass jar. When my kids were elementary school age, I would prep jars of grapes for them to have as self-serve snacks during the week.

Halved: 2 to 3 days in a glass food storage container or glass jar. I'd prep grapes this way when my youngest was a toddler.

Green Beans

Seasonality: Fresh green beans are available at US supermarkets nearly year-round. Peak season runs from May to September.

Shopping: Green beans aren't always green—you'll often find yellow, purple, and striped beans at farmers' markets. No matter the color, look for bright, smooth pods. Watch out for stiffness, wrinkles, or lumps—this can mean the beans are older or over-ripe. A telltale sign of freshness is that the beans snap easily when bent.

Prep and Storage

Washing: Place green beans in a colander and rinse with cool water. Then snap off the ends, pulling any hanging strings down the length of the pod. You can leave beans whole or cut them into smaller pieces before cooking.

Ethylene: Green beans have low ethylene production and medium ethylene sensitivity.

Optimal storage conditions: 40° to 45°F with 95% relative humidity

Whole (unwashed): I've seen a noticeable difference in shelf life for green beans from a farmers' market or CSA box compared to those from the supermarket. Shelf life will vary widely depending on how fresh the green beans were at time of purchase.

- **Farmers' market or CSA box:** 10 to 14 days in a plastic, paper, cotton, or linen bag in the crisper drawer. I've also had good results storing them in a paper bag on a middle shelf.

- **Supermarket:** 7 to 9 days in a plastic bag; 6 to 8 days in a cotton or linen bag in the crisper drawer or in a glass food storage container on a lower shelf

Chopped or sliced: 3 to 4 days in a glass food storage container or glass jar

Lightly steamed: 5 to 7 days in a glass food storage container or glass jar

Green Onions and Spring Onions

Seasonality: Green onions (aka scallions) are available in US supermarkets year-round, and their peak season runs from spring to summer. Spring onions are typically found at supermarkets and farmers' markets from May through June during their peak season, although they may be available earlier depending on your region.

Shopping: I like to focus on the roots of green onions and the bulbs of spring onions first to gauge freshness and plant health. Bright white bulbs and roots free from browning or excessive slime signal fresher stock. Then take a look at the green tops—they should be about 8 inches long. Avoid those with wilted or cracking tops.

Prep and Storage

Washing: Green onions are a veggie that I always like to wash immediately, even if I'm not going to use them right away. They have strong, sturdy layers that don't mind the extra moisture. Rinse bunches of green onions or spring onions under cool running water, using your fingers to pull off unwanted layers around the roots or bulbs. Pay special attention to getting water into the green tops, where sand and soil can often accumulate. (Alternatively, soak green onions or spring onions in cool water for 10 to 15 minutes before rinsing.) Gently dry with a dish towel.

Ethylene: Both green onions and spring onions have low ethylene production but high ethylene sensitivity.

Optimal storage conditions: 32°F with 95 to 100% relative humidity

Whole bunch (washed): 10 to 14 days, standing upright in a glass jar filled halfway with water and tented with a plastic bag. Be sure to really clean off broken or damaged layers near the bulbs and roots before placing them in water. After 4 or 5 days, change the water in the jar and remove any soggy layers from the onions. Because their roots are intact, you'll notice green onions and spring onions will continue to grow in your fridge when stored like this. Sometimes in a pinch I'll store my green onion roots in water in the fridge and let them build up again.

Chopped (large dice): 7 to 9 days in a glass food storage container or glass jar with little air exposure

Chopped (small dice): 5 to 7 days in a glass food storage container or glass jar, tightly packed, with little air exposure

Herbs

As a general rule, you want to keep fresh herbs—including basil, chives, dill, mint, parsley, rosemary, sage, thyme—separate from other produce and protected from moisture loss while not allowing excess moisture to build up and accelerate spoilage.

Prep and Storage

Basil

Optimal storage conditions: Basil is undoubtedly the most finicky of the soft herbs. With a preferred storage temperature of 50°F with 90% humidity, it's nearly impossible to reproduce ideal conditions in your home. Your best bet with basil is to use it quickly.

Unwashed:

- **Method 1:** 2 to 3 days in a glass jar filled halfway with water on the counter

- **Method 2:** 3 to 4 days in a dry glass jar with the lid only partially covering the jar opening on the counter

- **Method 3:** 3 to 4 days in a cotton or linen bag in a warmer area of your fridge (the crisper drawer or butter keeper on the door)

Chives

Optimal storage conditions: 32°F with 95 to 100% relative humidity

Whole (unwashed): 5 to 7 days in a glass food storage container. I've also had similar shelf life results storing chives in a linen bag in the crisper drawer.

Chopped: 2 to 3 days in a glass food storage container

Dill

Optimal storage conditions: 32°F with 95 to 100% relative humidity

Whole (unwashed): 7 to 9 days in a glass food storage container loosely covered with a paper napkin or paper towel and a tight-fitting lid. I've had similar shelf life results storing dill in a cotton or linen bag in the crisper drawer or leaving it in its original plastic clamshell in the butter keeper on the door.

Mint

Optimal storage conditions: 32°F with 95 to 100% relative humidity

Whole (unwashed): 7 to 9 days in a glass food storage container loosely covered with a paper napkin or paper towel and a tight-fitting lid. I've also had similar shelf life results storing mint in a cotton or linen bag in the crisper drawer or leaving it in the supermarket clamshell in the butter keeper on the door.

Chopped: 2 to 3 days in a glass food storage container. You'll notice some browning begin to occur where the leaves were cut toward the end of the shelf life.

Parsley

Optimal storage conditions: 32°F with 95 to 100% relative humidity

Whole (unwashed): 10 to 16 days standing upright in a glass jar filled halfway with water and tented with a plastic bag. Remove any leaves from the stem area of the bunch before placing it in the water. When you need to use some, simply tear a handful or two of leaves off the bunch (leaving the stems in the jar). After 4 or 5 days, change the water in the jar and remove any soggy leaves from the stem area.

Chopped: 4 to 6 days in a glass food storage container or glass jar with little air exposure. Pay special attention to drying the washed parsley as much as possible before chopping. Parsley will naturally dry out over this time.

Woody herbs (rosemary, sage, thyme)

Optimal storage conditions: 32°F with 90 to 95% relative humidity

Whole (unwashed): 7 to 10 days in a small cotton or linen bag inside a glass food storage container with a tight-fitting lid; 5 to 7 days in a plastic bag, plastic clamshell, or cotton or linen bag in the crisper drawer or in the butter keeper on the door. Do not wash until ready to use.

Kale

Seasonality: In recent years, fresh kale has been available year-round at US supermarkets. Kale is a cool-weather crop; peak season runs from November to April.

Types:

- **Curly kale** has tightly wound dark green or sometimes purple leaves. This is the type of kale you'll most often see at supermarkets.

- **Dinosaur (aka Tuscan or lacinato) kale** has large, crinkled blue-green leaves that are about 3 inches wide and slightly curved in along the edges.

- **Red or Red Russian kale** has red or purple stems and silvery-green to blue-green leaves. The leaves aren't crinkled or curly, but rather look like elongated oak leaves.

- **Redbor kale** has stems and curly leaves of a deep red to maroon color. Some variants will be entirely magenta or tinged with green.

Shopping: Smaller-leafed kale will be more tender and milder in flavor—great if you're planning to eat it raw. Look for moist, crisp, unwilted kale. Avoid bunches with tiny holes or yellowing or browning on the leaves, or browning on the stems, which can signal insect damage or decay.

Prep and Storage

Washing: I like to fill my sink with cool water and soak kale for 10 minutes, then rinse each leaf individually so I can examine them for possible cabbage aphid colonies. Aphids have a hankering for cruciferous veggies but are not a problem and will wash away with water.

Ethylene: Kale has very low ethylene production but high ethylene sensitivity.

Optimal storage conditions: 32°F with 95 to 100% relative humidity

Whole (unwashed):

- **Farmers' market or CSA box:** 10 to 14 days in a partially open plastic, cotton, or linen bag in the crisper drawer (if storing with high-ethylene-producing foods, keep the bag fully closed)

- **Supermarket:** 7 to 9 days in a plastic bag; 6 to 8 days in a cotton or linen bag in the crisper drawer

Chopped or torn by hand: 7 to 9 days in a glass food storage container or glass jar

Thinly sliced: 5 to 7 days in a glass food storage container or glass jar

Lightly steamed or sautéed: 7 to 9 days in a glass food storage container or glass jar

HOW TO TELL IF KALE HAS GONE BAD: The leaves will begin to wilt and turn pale green or yellow. The smell will change from a "green" cruciferous smell to a more intense sulfurous smell.

Leeks

Seasonality: Leeks are available year-round at US supermarkets. They are harvested twice a year: in early to midsummer and late fall to early winter. Peak seasons will vary based on region.

Shopping: Look for leeks that are mostly white and light green (as those are the edible parts of the plant). Stalks should be crisp and firm. Select smaller leeks for the best taste; aim for no more than 1½ inches in diameter. Watch out for leeks that are withered or have yellowed tops.

Prep and Storage

Washing: Leeks are grown in sandy soil. To remove as much of the soil as possible, slice them before washing. Cut off the root end, then slice the leek in half lengthwise and chop or slice. Place in a bowl of cold water, then agitate the leeks well. Drain in a colander.

Ethylene: Leeks have very low ethylene production and medium ethylene sensitivity.

Optimal storage conditions: 32°F with 95 to 100% relative humidity

Whole (unwashed): 10 to 14 days in a plastic bag in the crisper drawer; 7 to 9 days in a cotton or linen bag in the crisper drawer. If you don't have room to house whole leeks in the crisper, you can keep on a middle or lower shelf and spritz the bag lightly with water after 3 to 4 days.

Large slices: 7 to 9 days in a glass food storage container or glass jar with little air exposure

Thinly sliced: 5 to 7 days in a glass food storage container or glass jar, tightly packed, with little air exposure

Lettuce

I'm not going to lie—keeping salad greens hydrated while not introducing too much moisture and accelerating leaf breakdown is a delicate dance. Here's some guidance for ten varieties of lettuce: five that are commonly found at supermarkets throughout the year and five that are considered specialty types. Because each of you will have a distinct fridge and ambient environment in your home, I'm not going to include how long their shelf lives might be. Instead, I'll give you the storage methods that have worked best for me over the years.

Seasonality: Lettuce is a cool-season crop. That means it grows well in the spring and fall in most US regions and that seedlings can even tolerate a light frost. You'll enjoy lettuce year-round in the most temperate regions. In warmer regions, peak lettuce season will happen in the spring and fall. In cooler climates, peak season shifts to late spring through summer.

Types: Lettuce varieties are grouped into two broad categories: leaf lettuces and head lettuces. Leaf lettuces grow in clusters of wavy or frilly leaves. Head lettuces are round, with more tightly arranged leaves. Within each type are many varieties; some are delicate and others are sturdier.

Shopping: Start by assessing the leaves: Think lively and firm. It's also a good idea to look at the stem end: If the lettuce was harvested very recently, the cut end will be moist and slightly oozy. If it's overly brown or dry (although remember, some of that is inevitable), that signifies an older product. If you're buying organic (which I highly recommend), minor spotting or holes, especially on the outer leaves, is common and doesn't mean the lettuce is bad.

Prep and Storage

Washing: For delicate lettuces, you're going to get the longest shelf life by storing the lettuce unwashed. Sturdier varieties can handle washing before storage, but it's important to dry them off as much as possible to prevent the leaves from getting slimy.

Ethylene: As a general rule, lettuces have very low ethylene production but high ethylene sensitivity.

Optimal storage conditions: 32° to 34°F with 95 to 100% relative humidity. Lettuce storage is a challenge, and when it comes to shelf life, there's no more frustrating piece of produce. Lettuce is mostly water, and it's inherently fragile. The minute it's harvested, it starts to lose water, beginning the inevitable march toward wilting and slimy leaves. There's just no other fate available—you eat it before that happens or it perishes.

Butterhead Lettuces

These lettuce varieties (including butter, Boston, Bibb, and oakleaf) are characterized by a loose head and grass-green leaves. In recent years, red varieties have become popular. Bibb lettuce is a smaller, even more delicate variety of butter lettuce. Oakleaf lettuce is a type of butterhead lettuce whose leaves are distinctively lobed, with deep and distinct protrusions, like an oak leaf.

- **Shopping:** Butterhead lettuces are fragile varieties and their leaves wilt quickly. Select heads with unwilted, well-colored leaves with no signs of damage or yellowing. Typically, butterhead lettuces are sold packaged in plastic clamshells at the supermarket. If you can find heads with the roots still intact, you'll get longer shelf life.

- **Storage:** I like keeping butter lettuces in their clamshells on a lower fridge shelf (just above the crisper drawers). Alternatively, you can place it in a plastic bag in the crisper drawer (make a few holes in the bag or leave the top slightly open).

Iceberg Lettuce

This pale green lettuce forms a tight, compact head like cabbage.

- **Shopping:** It's all about selecting the ideal compact head—if you can press down on the head with moderate hand pressure, it's ideal. A very loose head indicates that the lettuce is immature but will still be tasty and nutritious; a very firm or hard head, on the other hand, is overmature and will likely have a shorter shelf life. It's important to note that the stem end of a head of iceberg lettuce may look brown—this discoloration is a natural result from harvesting and doesn't mean the head is too old.

- **Storage:** The iceberg lettuce you find at supermarkets comes ideally wrapped with a tight perforated plastic. The head can be stored in this original packaging in the crisper drawer and should keep for up to 2 weeks. If purchased from a farmers' market or received in a CSA delivery, you'll want to leave the lettuce unwashed and store it in a plastic bag in the crisper drawer (make a few holes in the bag or leave the top slightly open). I've also had good results storing iceberg lettuce in cotton or linen produce bags, which I spritz with water on days 1, 4, and 7 of storage.

Leaf Lettuces

This type of lettuce comprises a number of varieties that don't form heads, because the loosely packed leaves branch from a single central stalk or core. For this reason, leaf lettuces are generally more perishable than head varieties. They come in green and red colors, and the leaves may be either ruffled or smooth.

- **Storage Method 1:** Keep the lettuce unwashed and the leaves attached to the stalk or core. Wrap the head in a paper towel and place in a plastic bag (make a few holes in the bag or leave the top slightly open). Store in the crisper drawer.

- **Storage Method 2:** Separate the leaves and rinse under cool water. Lay the damp leaves on a dish towel and blot completely dry with another towel. Store in a glass food storage container with a tight-fitting lid.

Mixed Baby Greens

Also known as spring mix, this is a combination of different varieties of lettuce, kale, and spinach. The "baby" label simply indicates they were harvested earlier, typically 3 to 4 weeks after planting. The leaves are small and tender with a milder taste. Their main claim to fame is their convenience, as you can find bags and containers of prewashed mixed greens year-round at your local supermarket.

- **Shopping:** Mixed baby greens are sold in packages or loose. At the supermarket, it's common to see plastic bags or large plastic clamshells of mixed greens. At farmers' markets or bulk stores, you'll see open bulk bins of greens. A great tip is to pick up mixed greens toward the end of your shopping trip so you can get them home faster (this helps to reduce those annoying slimy leaves).

- **Washing:** Prewashed varieties are typically cleaned in a water-chlorine solution and stored in "breathable" plastic bags that are treated to maximize shelf life. I only recommend washing mixed greens that were purchased loose.

- **Storage:** I typically purchase mixed greens from Costco, where they are sold tightly packed into large plastic clamshells. Packing them so tightly can lead to slimy spots, so I like to give the greens more "breathing room" when I get them home by dividing them into several large glass food storage containers. This is also a great opportunity to remove any browning or slimy leaves. I arrange these on a lower fridge shelf, pulled toward the front of the fridge (to make sure they're away from the airflow source). If condensation buildup is an issue in your fridge, it's a good idea to lay a paper napkin or paper towel over the greens before closing the container so any moisture buildup on the lid doesn't lead to spoilage.

Romaine (or Cos) Lettuce

Romaine has long, deep-green leaves that form a loaf-shaped head. Some varieties develop a closed, compact head; others are more open. Romaine has a crisp texture and a strong, but not bitter, taste. Romaine is a hearty lettuce; I've frequently had it keep for over 3 weeks.

- **Shopping:** Look for romaine heads with closely bunched leaves that look fresh, and avoid those with brown or wilted leaves and soft or streaked leaf stems.

- **Storage Method 1:** Place romaine heads in a large plastic bag with some ventilation (make a few holes in the bag or leave the top slightly open). Store in the crisper drawer. I've noticed that whole heads do the best when stored upright.

- **Storage Method 2:** Separate the romaine leaves and arrange them loosely in a large glass food storage container with a tight-fitting lid. Store on one of the lower shelves in your fridge. You can use this storage method with either unwashed or washed romaine—just make sure to fully dry the leaves before storing.

Arugula

Also known as rocket or Italian cress, this peppery-tasting salad green has flat leaves with deep lobes. Older and larger leaves will have a more mustardy flavor.

- **Shopping:** Look for dry, firm, dark-green leaves, and avoid any wilted or wet leaves. Fresh arugula will have a peppery, sharp scent (much like its flavor), although this can be hard to discern when the leaves are bagged.

- **Storage:** Arugula is a delicate green. It tastes the best eaten within 5 days. I've had the best results storing it in a cotton or linen bag inside a perforated plastic bag in the crisper drawer; stored this way, it keeps for up to 10 days. You can also wrap the arugula leaves in paper napkins or paper towels to mimic this effect. I've also had excellent and consistent results storing arugula in glass food storage containers on a lower fridge shelf, pulled toward the front of the fridge (to make sure they're away from the airflow source). Arugula that's stored for too long or at too low a temperature will yellow, wilt, and develop brown spots.

Endive (aka White Chicory)

This pale salad green forms a small, cigar-shaped head with tightly packed leaves and has a slightly bitter flavor.

- **Shopping:** Look for endive heads that are crisp and brightly colored. If choosing Belgian endives, select heads with pale yellow-green tips. Avoid heads that are wilted or have browning.

- **Storage:** Wrap the whole endive in a paper napkin or paper towel and place in a perforated plastic bag in the crisper drawer. Placing the endive in a cotton or linen bag in lieu of the paper napkin/paper towel, then in a perforated plastic bag also works well. Both methods provide me with at least a week of storage. If the leaves look wilted toward the end of the week, soak them in a bowl of cold water to revive them!

Frisée

Frisée is not technically a lettuce, but in recent years, you may have seen it creeping onto salad plates. It is a leafy green related to endive and chicory. It grows into a head with a compact heart and frizzy, ripple-edged leaves that are green on the outer sections and lighter closer to the stem and stalk. Frisée's flavor is mildly bitter and peppery.

- **Storage:** Wrap the frisée head in a paper napkin or paper towel and place in a perforated plastic bag in the crisper drawer. Placing the frisée in a cotton or linen bag in lieu of the paper napkin/paper towel, then in a perforated plastic bag also works well. Both methods provide me with at least a week of storage.

Radicchio

Radicchio looks like a small red-and-white head of iceberg lettuce and can range in size from 2 to 5 inches in diameter. It has closely packed leaves that can be green, wine red, or magenta, with white veining.

- **Shopping:** Look for firm, brightly colored heads with crisp leaves. Watch out for damaged stem ends or browning leaves—signs of an older head.

- **Storage:** Wrap the unwashed radicchio head in a paper napkin or paper towel and place in a perforated plastic bag in the crisper drawer. Placing the radicchio in a cotton or linen bag in lieu of the paper napkin/paper towel, then in a perforated plastic bag also works well. If wilting occurs, soak the leaves in a bowl of cold water to revive them.

Watercress

Part of the mustard family of greens, watercress has a peppery flavor and is sold year-round at US supermarkets.

- **Shopping:** This delicate green is sold in trimmed bouquets. Look for perky, glossy, dark-green leaves and avoid any that are yellowing, wilting, or slimy. You can often find hydroponically grown watercress sold in hard plastic clamshells, with the root nub still in place.

- **Storage:** Hydroponic watercress stored in its plastic pack will keep for at least a week in your crisper drawer. Otherwise, I like to store watercress the same way I store soft herbs like cilantro and parsley: in a glass jar filled halfway with water and tented with a plastic bag, placed on a lower shelf and pulled toward the front of your fridge.

Melons

After they're harvested, melons won't get riper with age. That's why the struggle to find a ripe melon is so real. Your best bet for finding the sweetest, tastiest melons is to buy in-season varieties and carefully compare the one you choose to the other melons on display. Use the variety-specific shopping guidelines that follow to ferret out the best fruit.

Cantaloupe

Seasonality: Cantaloupe is frequently available in US supermarkets. Its peak season is from June till August (this can vary a bit based on region), and it is also frequently imported from South America.

Shopping: Like most melons, a good cantaloupe will feel heavy for its size. A good indicator of ripeness is to press with your thumb on the stem end and see if it gives a little. It's also a good idea, if you have the time, to gently press the cantaloupe all over to detect any squishy parts, which can mean it's overripe.

Prep and Storage

Ethylene: Cantaloupes have high ethylene production and medium ethylene sensitivity.

Optimal storage conditions: 36° to 41°F with 95% relative humidity

Whole (unwashed): If you have a not-yet-ready-to-slice cantaloupe, let it soften on your counter for 2 days (once harvested, the melon's sweetness is fixed, but the flesh will get softer and more fragrant). You can place it in a paper bag to soften it faster. Store a ripe cantaloupe in your fridge for just less than a week or a bit longer in the crisper drawer.

Halved (with seeds): 4 to 6 days on a lower shelf, with the cut side covered with plastic wrap. Leaving the seeds intact will help to retain moisture.

Sliced: 4 to 6 days in a glass food storage container

Large chunks: 4 to 6 days in a glass food storage container or glass jar, tightly packed, with little air exposure

Honeydew

Seasonality: Honeydew is available year-round in US supermarkets, with peak season running between June and October.

Shopping: Look for a honeydew that's firm but not too hard and that has a floral scent. Typically, as with all melons, the heavier it is for its size, the juicier it will be.

Prep and Storage

Ethylene: Honeydews have medium ethylene production and high ethylene sensitivity.

Optimal storage conditions: 41° to 50°F with 85 to 90% relative humidity

Whole (unwashed): Store the whole honeydew at room temperature for 2 to 4 days. Once sliced, wrap and refrigerate for up to 5 days. Can be stored on your counter if your ambient conditions are conducive. Otherwise, store in your crisper drawer or a lower fridge shelf until ready to cut or eat.

Sliced: 5 to 7 days in a glass food storage container

Large diced: 5 to 7 days in a glass food storage container or glass jar, tightly packed, with little air exposure

Watermelon

Seasonality: US watermelon season runs from May to September, although this can vary by region. Smaller watermelons imported from Mexico and South America are often available in supermarkets in the off season.

Shopping: Choose a watermelon that's heavy for its size. Make sure to find the "ground spot," a creamy-yellow or straw-colored spot on the rind where the melon rested on the soil in the field, which can help you determine the melon's ripeness. During the growing process, these spots start out white and gradually change color as the sugar content increases. When they're gold, that means the watermelons have fully matured and are ready to be harvested.

Prep and Storage

Ethylene: Watermelon has very low ethylene production but high ethylene sensitivity.

Optimal storage conditions: 50° to 59°F with 90% relative humidity

Whole (unwashed): Can be stored on your counter if the ambient conditions are conducive. If your home conditions are warmer than 59°F, don't leave the watermelon out for more than 2 days before cutting up the melon for eating or longer storage in the fridge. I frequently store whole mini watermelons in the fridge with no adverse changes in flavor or texture.

Sliced: 5 to 7 days in a glass food storage container

Large dice: 5 to 7 days in a glass food storage container or glass jar, tightly packed, with little air exposure

Microgreens

Microgreens are simply the seedlings of edible plants (especially vegetables and herbs) harvested early (around 1 to 3 weeks, depending on the plant). The difference between a microgreen and a sprout is that microgreens are grown in soil or a growing medium, whereas sprouts are grown with water only. With sprouts, you get to eat the seeds; with microgreens, you eat the stem and leaves.

Seasonality: Microgreens are typically grown indoors and are not seasonal.

Shopping: Microgreens are becoming more readily available at supermarkets. I typically find cilantro, broccoli, radish, and mixed microgreens stocked in the refrigerated produce section.

Prep and Storage

Washing: Microgreens are extremely delicate and should not be washed until just before you plan to eat them. I grab a handful from their container and rinse them in my hand under cool water, then pat dry with a dish towel.

Unwashed: 6 to 8 days in their original plastic clamshell in the crisper drawer; 7 to 9 days in a glass jar or glass food storage container, loosely packed, pulled up toward the front of the fridge. If using a storage container, wrap the microgreens in a paper napkin or place in small cotton or linen produce bag before putting them in the container. No matter which storage method you use, it's a good idea to pull out any wilting or excessively wet leaves before long-term storage. Microgreens are susceptible to turning slimy like mixed baby greens.

Mushrooms

Seasonality: Modern mushroom cultivation techniques mean common varieties are available in US supermarkets year-round. Almost half the nation's commercial mushroom crop is grown in Pennsylvania; the fungi are grown in large ventilated "barns," which produce four to six harvests every year. Most wild mushrooms only appear in fall; morel season occurs in the spring.

Shopping: Look for mushrooms that are plump with a fresh, smooth appearance—not dried out.

Prep and Storage

Washing: It's always best to store your mushrooms unwashed. When I'm ready to prepare the mushrooms, I place them in a colander and rinse them with cool water, then lay them out on a dish towel and pat dry.

Ethylene: Mushrooms have very low ethylene production and medium ethylene sensitivity.

Optimal storage conditions: 32°F with 90% relative humidity

Whole (unwashed): The full storage life after harvest is 14 days but will vary depending on how the mushrooms are packaged. Stored in their original plastic packaging, they will keep for 5 to 7 days—this will vary depending on how soon after harvest the mushrooms were purchased. Keep the mushrooms away from direct airflow sources, as this can dry them out, and do not store them in your crisper drawers, as the combination of plastic packaging and the more humid environment of the crisper is too moist for mushrooms and will result in slime. Stored in a paper bag in the crisper drawer or away from an airflow source, they will keep for 7 to 9 days, especially if you purchased them loose.

Large slices or dice: 3 to 4 days loosely arranged in a glass food storage container or glass jar

Thinly sliced or minced: 2 to 3 days loosely arranged in a glass food storage container or glass jar

Sautéed or roasted: 7 to 9 days in a glass food storage container or glass jar, well packed, with little air exposure

Onions

Seasonality: Yellow, white, and red onions are available year-round in the US, but there are two main harvesttimes: Spring/summer onions are available from March to August. This harvest produces onions with thinner skin, a milder flavor, and higher water content. The fall/winter harvest runs from August to May. This harvest produces onions with thicker, darker-colored skins, lower water content (which leads to a longer shelf life), and more pungent flavors. Sweet onion varieties, such as Vidalia and Walla Walla, are available from late April through August. Onions have to cure for 2 to 4 weeks after harvest, and commercial crops are cured under tightly controlled conditions. When housed in their optimal conditions (with artificial climate controls), onions can be stored for up to 8 months.

Shopping: Choose onions that are round and firm; avoid ones that are bruised or moldy. I always look for red and yellow onions with the darkest color skins; these are more consistently the tastiest.

Prep and Storage

Ethylene: Onions have very low ethylene production and low ethylene sensitivity.

Optimal storage conditions: 32°F with 65 to 70% relative humidity

Whole: Store whole onions in a cool, dark, well-ventilated place for use within 4 weeks. They store well with garlic because they have the same ethylene profile. I store my onions in wooden storage bins in my pantry cart that are lidded but not airtight, which allows for airflow. Keeping the light away is critical to avoid sprouting. If your indoor climate is unusually humid or hot, you're best off buying new onions weekly and prepping them to keep in the fridge. Storing whole onion bulbs may cause sprouting, but if you use them within 7 to 9 days and store them outside of the crisper drawer, in the drier part of the fridge, it shouldn't be a problem. You can also store peeled whole onions in an airtight container and keep in the fridge for 10 to 14 days.

Halved: 7 to 9 days in a small glass food storage container, glass jar, plastic bag, or covered with plastic wrap

Thick slices or large dice: 5 to 7 days in a glass food storage container or glass jar

Thinly sliced or small dice: 3 to 5 days in a glass food storage container or glass jar

Sautéed or roasted: 7 to 9 days in a glass food storage container, tightly packed, with little air exposure. For longer shelf life, push the container back toward the airflow source.

Pears

Types: There are two types of pears, European and Asian, and many varieties of each type. For our purposes, we'll focus on the varieties most common in US supermarkets.

- **European pears:** These pears have a lower water content and for that reason are ideal for cooking. **Bartlett** is the variety most common in the US and is in season from August until December. Bartlett pears come in two colors—green and red—and have a classic pear flavor with a buttery-soft texture. **Bosc** pears are available from late September to April. They have a longer neck and bronze-colored skin, and their crispy, juicy flesh is sweet, with hints of cinnamon. Named for a region in France, **Anjou** pears arrive in markets in late September or early October and are available many months of the year. These egg-shaped red or green pears have a mild flavor and a very firm texture, which makes them ideal for cooking and baking.

- **Asian pears:** Depending on your region, Asian pear season may begin as early as July and last until winter, reaching their peak in September and October. Also known as apple pears or sand pears, Asian pears have a shape and texture similar to an apple, with a high water content and exceptionally refreshing flavor.

Shopping: The longer European-variety pears ripen on the tree, the grainier their texture becomes, so the key is to select unripe pears and allow them to ripen at home. Select pears that are slightly firm, without soft spots or cuts. You'll shop a bit differently for Asian pears, which are harvested ripe and are ready to eat when purchased. The good news is, they have an extremely long shelf life in the fridge.

Prep and Storage

Ethylene: Both European and Asian pears have high ethylene production and high ethylene sensitivity.

Optimal storage conditions:

- **Asian pears:** 34°F with 90 to 95% relative humidity

- **European pears:** 29° to 31°F with 90 to 95% relative humidity

Whole (European): Allow to ripen on your countertop. Test for ripeness by pressing your thumb against the stem area and feeling for some give. European pears have a tendency to quickly go bad after ripening, so once ripe, transfer them to your crisper drawer to get a few more days of shelf life.

Whole (Asian): Up to 3 months in the crisper, away from ethylene-producing or -sensitive foods. They can also be placed in a lidded glass or plastic food storage container if you don't have space in your crisper. If most of my food is stored in glass containers, I'll leave my Asian pears out on a lower shelf toward the front of the fridge if I plan to eat them within the week. For longer than a week storage, you can keep them in a plastic produce bag or zip-top bag on a lower shelf in the fridge.

Peas

Seasonality: All pea varieties are available year-round (fresh or frozen) in US super-markets. Domestic peas are in season from early spring to early summer, with imports from South America filling in any production gaps; you may see fresh peas at your farmers' market during a short window in early spring. Snap peas are more tolerant of hot weather than garden peas; their season lasts until about early July, or until temperatures reach the mid-80s in a given region.

Types:

- **Garden peas:** Also known as English peas, green peas, or just plain old "peas" (when found in the frozen section). They grow in pods but must be shucked before eating, as the pods are inedible.

- **Snow peas:** Also known as Chinese peas or mangetouts (their French name, which means "eat all," since you eat them pod and all). Snow peas are instantly recognizable because they have an almost entirely flat, edible pod. They can be eaten raw or cooked, but are most commonly cooked.

- **Snap peas:** These can be differentiated by their pod shape, which is slightly more cylindrical than that of English peas. Snap peas have edible pods like snow peas but round, plump peas like garden peas. Sugar snap peas, the most common variety, are a hybrid of garden peas and snow peas; have thick, crisp, and crunchy pods; and can be eaten raw or cooked.

Shopping: Look for plump, firm, brightly colored pods. Snap peas typically have lighter-green areas of pod damage, which is perfectly normal and doesn't mean they are bad. Peas are a great vegetable to buy frozen because their sugars turn into starch the longer they sit after harvest.

Prep and Storage

Washing: I place pods in a large colander and rinse them in cool running water when I'm ready to use or prep them.

Ethylene: All types of pod peas have very low ethylene production and medium ethylene sensitivity.

Optimal storage conditions: 32°F with 90 to 98% relative humidity

All types, whole/in the pod (unwashed): 8 to 10 days in their original bag (or other plastic bag) in the crisper drawer; 8 to 14 days loosely arranged in a glass food storage container or glass jar, pulled toward the front of the fridge; 6 to 8 days in a cotton or linen bag in the crisper drawer

Snow peas or snap peas, chopped: 6 to 8 days in a glass food storage container or glass jar, packed, with little air exposure

Garden peas, shucked: 7 to 9 days in a glass food storage container or glass jar, pulled to the front of the shelf

Pineapple

Seasonality: Pineapple is available year-round in US supermarkets, with peak season running from March through July. One of the most disappointing discoveries for me after returning from our family trip to Hawaii was that Hawaiian-grown pineapples are not sold in supermarkets on the US mainland. The state's pineapple industry currently exists primarily to satisfy local demands. The major fruit companies pulled out of Hawaii between the early 1990s and 2008. Now you'll mostly find pineapples are imported from Costa Rica and other Central American or South American countries.

Shopping: Pineapples don't continue to sweeten and ripen after they're harvested. Choose a pineapple with a yellow-gold color that reaches as far up toward the leaves as possible, because the sweetest part of the pineapple is at the bottom. Look for a large, plump pineapple that's slightly soft to the touch, with crisp, dark green leaves. Watch out for wrinkling or soft skin or dry, browning leaves, as this means the fruit is deteriorating.

Prep and Storage

Ethylene: Pineapples have both low ethylene production and low ethylene sensitivity.

Optimal storage conditions: 45° to 55°F with 85 to 90% relative humidity

Whole (unwashed): 3 to 5 days on your kitchen counter. If your ambient conditions are too hot, I recommend cutting it promptly and storing the chunks in the fridge. If I know I'm going to store pineapple chunks chopped in the fridge, I like to place the whole pineapple in the fridge the day before to cool down the flesh before chopping.

Chunks: 5 to 7 days in a glass food storage container or glass jar, pulled toward the front of the fridge. The more natural pineapple juice you can store the chunks with, the better.

Frozen: 3 to 5 months. If you have excess fresh pineapple, arrange it on a baking sheet lined with parchment paper and freeze it overnight, then transfer the frozen pineapple to a plastic storage container with a tight-fitting lid and store in the freezer.

Potatoes and Sweet Potatoes

Seasonality: Available year-round in US supermarkets, most potatoes are harvested in September and October, with new potatoes in season from April to July.

Types: There are thousands of varieties of potatoes grown around the world, but here are the types and varieties you're most likely to find at US supermarkets.

- **White:** The most common of this variety is the russet potato, which has a long body, rough skin, and fluffy white flesh. These are considered "starchy" potatoes.

- **Red:** Shorter and rounder than russets, with red skin. Their flesh can be either white or yellow. Red potatoes are called "waxy" potatoes because they have less starch and hold their shape better when cooked than starchy potatoes do.

- **Yellow:** Sometimes called creamer potatoes, these are smaller, rounder, and have a thinner skin than russets. Yellow potatoes cook quickly and have buttery-tasting flesh. Yellow potatoes fall in between starchy and waxy potatoes with a medium starch level.

- **Sweet potatoes and yams:** Most commonly orange-skinned and -fleshed, but there are also sweet potatoes with pale copper/tan skin and white flesh, red skin with dry white flesh, and purple skin and flesh. Their flavor profiles vary, but they are all more slender than a potato and have tapered ends. Although "yam" is a common term for sweet potatoes, real yams have dark, rough, barklike skin and dry, starchy flesh; they are rarely seen in US supermarkets.

- **Fingerling potatoes:** You'll often find small bags of multicolored fingerling potatoes in the produce department. Fingerling potatoes are a full-grown specific variety of potato. They get their name because they're long and slender and about the size of a finger. They are waxy like red potatoes.

- **Purple/blue fingerlings:** These are sometimes found at farmers' markets and increasingly at supermarkets.

- **New potatoes:** Not a variety of potato, new potatoes are baby potatoes of any variety that are harvested before fully mature. This is a result of farmers thinning a normal potato crop—making room in the soil for the remaining potatoes to reach their full size. New potatoes have very delicate skins and a similar shape to fingerlings. They have a creamier and sweeter flavor than normal potatoes. Because they are more delicate, they don't store nearly as well as their full-grown counterparts.

Shopping: For all potatoes, I try to buy organic whenever possible because I like to eat the skins. Choose potatoes that are firm, with no soft or dark spots. Avoid sprouting or green-tinged potatoes, as they can contain toxic alkaloids that develop when exposed to light. When selecting sweet potatoes, remember that the nutrition content is directly linked to the intensity of its skin and flesh color.

Prep and Storage

Washing: I like to fill my sink with cool water and allow the potatoes to soak for at least 20 minutes, then scrub the skins with a dish towel to remove any stubborn dirt or dust.

Ethylene: Potatoes have very low ethylene production and medium ethylene sensitivity.

Optimal storage conditions:

- New (or "early crop") potatoes: 50° to 59°F with 90 to 95% relative humidity

- Mature (or "late crop") potatoes: 40° to 46°F with 95 to 98% relative humidity

- Sweet potatoes: 55° to 59°F with 90% to 95% relative humidity

Whole, mature (unwashed): 1 to 2 months in a cool, dry place

Whole, new (unwashed): 5 to 7 days on the counter in a darker area of the kitchen

Chopped: Up to 2 days in a glass food storage container or glass jar filled with water in the fridge. I sometimes chop potatoes like this when I'm batch prepping meals. Note that when you store or soak potatoes in water, it naturally removes some of their starch. Storing longer than 2 days like this can affect their taste.

Steamed or boiled, skin on (whole or large pieces): 7 to 9 days in a glass food storage container or glass jar

Baked or roasted, skin on (whole or wedges): 9 to 12 days in a glass food storage container or glass jar. Baked sweet potatoes are one of my favorite foods to prep ahead, because they keep so long in the fridge.

Radishes

Seasonality: Radishes are a cool-weather crop. Classic red radishes are available at US supermarkets nearly year-round, with peak season running from late winter to spring. Specialty varieties will have varying peak seasons. For example, watermelon radishes peak in both the late fall and the spring.

Shopping: Look for plump, firm bulbs and crisp, bright green leaves (if attached). The greens are edible, but some varieties have a fuzzy texture that may be off-putting.

Prep and Storage

Washing: When ready to eat or prepare, soak them in a bowl of cool water and wipe off any stubborn spots with a dish towel.

Ethylene: Radishes have very low ethylene production and low ethylene sensitivity.

Optimal storage conditions: 32°F with 95 to 100% relative humidity

Whole (unwashed), greens trimmed: Remove the greens before storing radishes to prevent nutrients and water from leaching into the leaves from the roots.

- **Method 1:** 2 to 3 weeks in a glass food storage container filled with water, pushed back near an airflow source in your fridge. Change the water every 5 to 7 days. If you plan on eating these within 2 weeks, they do not need to be pushed back on the shelf.

- **Method 2:** 10 to 12 days in a glass food storage container, without water

- **Method 3:** Up to 2 weeks in a cotton or linen produce bag in the crisper drawer or in a glass food storage container on a lower shelf, pushed toward the front of the fridge

Large slices: 8 to 10 days in a glass food storage container or glass jar filled with water, or 6 to 8 days without water (some drying out may occur toward the end of their shelf life)

Thinly sliced or diced: 6 to 8 days in a glass food storage container or glass jar filled with water, or 5 to 7 days without water (some drying out may occur toward the end of their shelf life)

Greens (unwashed): 5 days in a plastic bag in the crisper drawer. They will keep a bit longer set upright in a glass jar filled halfway with water (removing any lower leaves so they are not submerged in the water) and tented with a plastic bag, pulled up near the front of the fridge.

Spinach

Seasonality: Fresh spinach is available at US supermarkets nearly year-round, with two peak seasons running from March through May and September through October. The fall season is when spinach is the freshest and has the best flavor. California, Arizona, New Jersey, and Texas grow 98% of the commercial fresh market spinach in the US.

Types: There are four types of spinach available in US supermarkets: smooth-leaf, savoy, semi-savoy, and baby spinach. Smooth-leaf has flat, unwrinkled, spade-shaped leaves, with a mild taste. Savoy has crinkled, curly, dark green leaves with a springy texture. Semi-savoy is similar in texture to savoy but is not as crinkled in appearance. Baby spinach is just spinach that's been harvested early. It's more delicate in flavor and texture than mature spinach and is ideal for raw salads because the stems are fine enough that they do not need to be removed.

Shopping: Choose spinach that has vibrant deep green leaves and stems, with no signs of yellowing. The leaves should look fresh and tender, not wilted or bruised. You'll typically find mature spinach sold in bunches and baby spinach sold in bags or plastic containers.

Prep and Storage

Washing: I don't wash spinach before storing it because it can be difficult to get it fully dry before putting it into the fridge, and excess moisture will cause it to slime. I also don't wash prewashed baby spinach—this is a personal preference. When I'm ready to eat or prepare fresh spinach, I rinse it under cool water, then spin it dry in my salad spinner.

Ethylene: Spinach has very low ethylene production but high ethylene sensitivity.

Optimal storage conditions: 32°F with 95 to 100% relative humidity

Mature spinach bunch (unwashed): 3 to 5 days in a loose plastic bag in the crisper drawer—you can add a napkin or paper towel to the bag if condensation is an issue in your fridge.

Baby spinach (prewashed): 7 to 9 days placed loosely into large glass food storage containers and stored on one of the lower shelves in the fridge. Pick out and discard any yellowing or slimy leaves before storing. I typically buy a large clamshell from Costco and separate it into three or four glass containers. At certain times of year, I've been able to keep baby spinach fresh for over 2 weeks with this method!

Mature spinach, cut: No more than 24 hours stored loosely in a glass food storage container or glass jar. I will sometimes cut spinach and store it overnight for batch cooking the next day.

Blanched: 7 to 9 days in a glass food storage container or glass jar, packed, with little air exposure

Stone Fruit

Seasonality: Specific seasonality varies wildly depending on the stone fruit variety. Generally, stone fruits—such as apricots, nectarines, peaches, plums, and pluots—are at their peak season from June to September and readily available at US supermarkets during the summer months.

Shopping: Buy organic when possible. And if you're looking for the best flavor, the key is to purchase locally grown stone fruits. They develop their flavor, perfume, and sweetness on the tree—which makes good stone fruit harder to transport over long distances.

Prep and Storage

Washing: I don't wash stone fruit until just before I'm ready to eat it; simply rinse under cool water.

Ethylene: All the stone fruits covered here have medium ethylene production and medium ethylene sensitivity.

Optimal storage conditions: 31° to 32°F with 90 to 95% relative humidity

Whole (unwashed): If the fruit is still firm, store it on your kitchen counter on a platter. Test for ripeness by pressing in right around the stem; if the flesh gives a bit, it's good to go. If you have stone fruit that's ripening too quickly, place it in the crisper drawer to get a few more days of shelf life. If you want to slow down ripening overall, store in the fridge crisper bins just after purchasing. The truth is, stone fruits are highly perishable.

Cut: No longer than 24 to 36 hours in a glass food storage container or glass jar (I only know this because I used to make my kid's lunches the day before). Make sure your container fits as close as possible to the amount of fruit you're storing.

FREEZING STONE FRUIT: Slice the fruit, arrange it on a baking sheet lined with parchment paper, and freeze it overnight. Then transfer the frozen stone fruit to a freezer storage container with a tight-fitting lid and store in the freezer for up to 3 months.

Summer Squash

Seasonality: Zucchini is available at US supermarkets nearly year-round, but the peak season, from June to late August, is the same for all summer squash varieties, which include crookneck, pattypan, and yellow squash.

Types:

- **Crookneck squash:** Usually yellow, this squash has a bulbous bottom that turns thin and curved at the top—they look like swan necks to me. Some varieties will have a warty, bumpy skin. In general, crookneck squash has a mild flavor with a tougher skin for summer squash. It should be harvested at 5 to 6 inches or less in length.

- **Pattypan squash:** Also known as scalloped squash or "UFO squash," because its squat, flat-bottomed shape has a flying-saucer-like appearance. Pattypan has a tougher skin and holds up well to cooking.

- **Yellow squash:** This summer squash has a signature bright yellow skin with a tapered top and a bulbous bottom. Its flesh has a texture very similar to zucchini, with a creamy, spongy interior.

- **Zucchini:** Mostly green, but can also be yellow and sometimes dark green with pale green stripes. While yellow squash has smooth, rounded skin, zucchini has straight, flattened sides and thin skin. Its flavor is slightly sweet.

Shopping: Larger squash tend to be less flavorful and more fibrous, with larger seeds. Aim for small to medium-length squashes (6 to 8 inches long), which typically have better flavor.

Prep and Storage

Washing: I only wash summer squash when I'm ready to prep or cook it. Place a few squash in a large colander and rinse with cool water.

Ethylene: All summer squash have low ethylene production and medium ethylene sensitivity.

Optimal storage conditions: 45° to 50°F with 95% relative humidity

Whole (unwashed): 8 to 10 days in a loose plastic bag in the crisper drawer—you can add a napkin or paper towel to the bag if condensation is an issue in your fridge; 7 to 9 days in a cotton or linen bag in the crisper drawer. Alternatively, if you don't have space in your crisper, you can store summer squash whole in a glass food storage container on a lower fridge shelf, pulled toward the front of the fridge.

Large dice: 5 to 7 days in a glass food storage container or glass jar

Spiralized or thinly sliced on a mandoline: 4 to 6 days stored loosely in a glass food storage container or glass jar

Swiss Chard

Seasonality: Chard is available nearly year-round in US supermarkets and farmers' markets because most species of chard produce three or more harvests, and it does well in both cool and hot climates. Peak season is July through November. Chard can be harvested young while its leaves are tender (you'll often find these leaves in mixed baby greens), or after maturing, when they are larger and have slightly tougher stems.

Types: The most common varieties are ruby chard, rhubarb chard, and rainbow chard. Ruby chard has bright red stalks and deep red veins in green leaves, while rhubarb chard has dark green leaves with a reddish stalk and a stronger flavor. Rainbow chard are other colorful chard varieties bunched together. The stalk colors may be pink, orange, red, yellow, purple, white with red stripes, or ivory with pink stripes.

Shopping: Look for crisp, strong, brightly colored stalks that aren't soft or wobbly. Tip the chard vertically to test the strength of the stems—this is a great indicator of freshness. Then check the stem cut for moisture—more moisture and less browning means the bunch is fresher. Avoid bunches with wilting, yellowing, or browning leaves.

Prep and Storage

Washing: I like to fill my sink with cool water and soak the chard for at least 10 minutes, then rinse the chard and remove any stubborn spots with a washcloth.

Ethylene: Swiss chard has very low ethylene production but high ethylene sensitivity.

Optimal storage conditions: 32°F with 95 to 100% relative humidity

Whole (unwashed):

- **Method 1:** Up to 7 days in a plastic bag, with the leaves wrapped in a paper towel. Store in the crisper drawer or on a lower fridge shelf, pulled up to the front of the fridge.

- **Method 2:** Separate the stalks from the leaves. Store the stalks in a glass jar with 2 inches of water at the bottom; tent the tops with a plastic bag. Rinse the leaves and wrap them in a cotton or linen dish towel and store in the crisper drawer or on a lower fridge shelf pulled up to the front of the fridge. Stored this way, leaves and stems will keep for up to 7 days; check on the leaves after 3 days and spritz with water if needed to keep them moist (especially if they're stored outside the crisper drawer).

- **Method 3:** Stand the bunch (with stems and leaves attached) in a 1-quart glass jar filled halfway with water; tent the top with a large plastic bag. Store toward the back of your fridge (to avoid spills—depending on the size of the chard, this option could require a shelf with lots of vertical room). During peak season, chard will keep for up 14 days with this method; change the water on day 4 or 5.

Leaves (washed): 4 to 6 days rolled in a kitchen towel or wrapped in linen produce bag and placed in the crisper drawer or a lower fridge shelf (see photos on pages 57 and 59).

Leaves, stemmed (washed): 5 to 7 days, cut with a sharp knife and packed loosely in a large glass food storage container with a tight-fitting lid.

Stems (washed): Use a sharp knife to cut the stems to fit inside a 1-quart or 1-pint widemouthed glass jar; fill the jar halfway with water and seal the lid tightly. Stored this way, the stems will keep for 7 to 9 days; change the water after about 4 days.

Stems, diced (washed): 4 to 6 days stored loosely in a glass food storage container or glass jar with little air exposure

Tomatoes

Seasonality: Thanks to commercial greenhouse growing operations and imports, tomatoes are available year-round in US supermarkets. But their peak season runs from May through October, with some variation depending on your region.

Types: There are over ten thousand varieties of tomatoes, but here are the types you're most likely to encounter at the supermarket or farmers' market:

- **Heirloom:** These can be large or small and have an incredibly complex taste and often a lower water content. The larger varieties have characteristically irregular shapes. Heirloom varieties get their name because the seeds have been passed down for generations without hybridization. They come in beautiful colors like green, yellow, purple, black, and striped.

- **Beefsteak:** Very large and bright red. Also known as "slicers," these are the juicy, meaty-textured tomatoes you're most likely to find on your restaurant burger or sandwich.

- **Plum (Roma):** These egg-shaped, thick-skinned, medium-size tomatoes can be red or yellow. They have fewer seeds, lower water content, higher acid content, and chewy flesh. Sometimes called Italian plums, paste tomatoes, or processing tomatoes, plum tomatoes are the variety most used for making tomato sauces and tomato paste.

- **Cherry:** Generally, the smaller the tomato fruit, the higher the sugar content. Cherry tomatoes are juicy and sweet and have thin skins. You'll find them in red, yellow, and orange.

- **Grape:** Similar in size and shape to grapes, these oblong tomatoes have thicker skins than cherry tomatoes and are about half their size. They have a high sugar content, and their flesh is meatier and less watery than that of cherry tomatoes. Popular varieties include Sweet 100 and Super Sweet 100.

Shopping: I always try to buy organic fresh tomatoes because I always eat the skin. Look for tomatoes that are firm, smooth, and brightly colored, without blemishes or bruises. Tomatoes on the vine tend to have a longer shelf life than loose tomatoes, especially when it comes to larger tomatoes.

Prep and Storage

Washing: Rinse in cool water, using a colander for smaller varieties, just before eating or cooking.

Ethylene: Mature but unripe tomatoes have very low ethylene production but high ethylene sensitivity. Ripe tomatoes have high ethylene production but low ethylene sensitivity.

Optimal storage conditions:

- Unripe mature tomatoes: 50° to 55°F with 90 to 95% relative humidity

- Ripe tomatoes: 46° to 50°F with 85 to 90% relative humidity

A NOTE ABOUT STORING TOMATOES IN THE FRIDGE: Tomatoes can only ripen at room temperature, and it's undeniable that they have the best taste and texture when stored at room temperature, too. But I'm not fully on board with the general consensus that tomatoes have no place in the fridge. This is especially the case with smaller varieties like grape tomatoes. Once ripened, grape tomatoes store very well in the fridge—I've seen no difference in texture or taste. I presume this is because they have thicker skin that protects the flesh against the cooler temperature.

I do agree that refrigerating larger tomato varieties can often result in a mealy texture and altered taste, but usually only after prolonged storage (longer than 4 or 5 days). If you have very ripe tomatoes that you can't eat right away, storing them in the fridge for 2 to 3 days will not ruin them. I recommend housing them in a glass food storage container with a tight-fitting lid on a lower fridge shelf.

Grape tomatoes (washed): 7 to 9 days in a glass food storage container or glass jar, pulled toward the front of the fridge.

Diced: 2 to 3 days, depending on the variety, in a glass food storage container or glass jar with very little air exposure. Adding lemon or lime juice can extend shelf life to 4 to 6 days.

HOW TO RIPEN TOMATOES FASTER: Place unripe tomatoes and a ripe apple in a brown paper bag (you can punch a few holes in it) and set aside on your countertop for 3 to 4 days. The apple's high ethylene production will help accelerate the tomatoes' ripening.

Turnips

Seasonality: Turnips are a cool-weather crop and have a short growing season. They are available at US supermarkets nearly year-round, with peak season running from October through March.

Shopping: It's important to look for the right size turnip for your needs. If you're planning to eat them raw or lightly steamed, select turnips that are on the small side (less than 3 inches wide). Smaller turnips are younger and more tender than mature turnips and have a mild taste. Larger, more mature turnips are more suitable for mashing or cooking in soups or stews.

Prep and Storage

Washing: Because turnips are root vegetables and grown mostly underground, I like to give them a good wash. Fill your sink with warm water and scrub off any stubborn dirt with a brush. Rinse turnip greens in cool running water and dry them thoroughly before storing or eating.

Ethylene: Turnips have very low ethylene production and low ethylene sensitivity.

Optimal storage conditions: 32°F with 95% relative humidity

Whole (unwashed): Up to 3 weeks in a plastic bag in the crisper drawer, or up to 2 weeks in a cotton or linen produce bag—especially if you periodically spritz them with water. Remove the turnip greens before storing, as they pull moisture from the root and decrease shelf life.

Greens (washed and dried well): 3 to 4 days placed loosely in a plastic bag—you can add a napkin or paper towel to the bag, if needed, to absorb excessive condensation; 4 to 6 days in a glass food storage container on a lower shelf, pulled toward the front of the fridge

Root (young and small), sliced (washed): 5 to 7 days in a glass food storage container or glass jar with little air exposure; you can store them in water as you would carrots or radishes to prevent any drying

Root, diced (washed): 5 to 7 days in a glass storage container or jar filled with water, or 2 to 3 days in a glass food storage container or glass jar, packed, with little air exposure

Winter Squash

Seasonality: Winter squash is harvested in late summer and early fall. Peak season is generally considered October and November, but you'll find them available at US supermarkets through the winter months as they store so well.

Types: These are the most common varieties of winter squash you're likely to encounter at your supermarket or local farmers' market.

- **Acorn squash:** Smaller in size for a winter squash and easy to recognize by their ridges and squat acorn shape. Their thick green-and-orange skin is edible. The flesh is a bit more watery than other varieties, with a yellow-orange color and a mild, sweet, nutty flavor.

- **Butternut squash:** Has a characteristic pear shape with a smooth, tan-colored rind. The flesh is bright orange, with few seeds, and has a nutty, sweet flavor (it's actually the sweetest tasting of all winter squash). Butternut squash has very tough skin that's often removed before cooking.

- **Delicata squash:** Also known as sweet potato squash, delicata squash is personally my favorite type of winter squash! Delicata are small and cylindrical in shape, with edible light yellow skin striped in green. The flesh is yellow-orange, with a creamy texture and mild flavor that tastes like a cross between very fresh corn and a sweet potato.

- **Kabocha squash:** Has a short, round body with a turned-out base and a dull, dark green rind that can sometimes have small lumps. The soft flesh is bright yellow-orange and has a sweet, nutty, pumpkinlike flavor. Kabocha are often peeled before cooking.

- **Red kuri squash:** Has orange skin and a teardrop shape. The flesh is creamy and yellow and tastes very similar to chestnuts. The skin is very hard but thin, so it is edible once cooked, though most people peel kuri squash before cooking.

- **Spaghetti squash:** This is a favorite of the low-carb set. Spaghetti squash has a cylindrical shape with yellow to cream-colored skin. It gets its name from its flesh, which is stringy and noodlelike once cooked, with a light, nutty flavor and a chewy, tender texture. This squash is not sweet.

- **Pumpkin:** Smaller "sugar pumpkins" are the varieties used for cooking. They have a round, bright-orange body, and their orange flesh has a sweet, earthy taste. Pumpkins should be peeled before eating.

Shopping: Look for hard, unblemished, uncracked, and colorful rinds; the squash should feel heavy for its size—this signifies a thick wall of edible flesh inside. Winter squash rinds don't always look pretty; just make sure to avoid any with distinct signs of decay.

Prep and Storage

Washing: I typically wipe down my winter squash with a washcloth dipped in a mixture of hot water and lemon juice just before I'm ready to prepare them.

Ethylene: Winter squash have low ethylene production and medium ethylene sensitivity.

Optimal storage conditions: 54° to 59°F with 50 to 70% relative humidity

Whole (unwashed): 2 to 3 months in a cool, dry place. Winter squash is an ambient storage superstar. But the big caveat is that your squash's particular shelf life will decrease if the ambient environment is warmer. In hot, humid climates, they will keep for up to 1 month if stored in a cool, dry part of your kitchen.

Peeled, seeded, and cubed (raw): 7 to 9 days in a glass food storage container or glass jar in the refrigerator

Pantry and Supplemental Storage

I know that this book is all about your fridge, but the rest of your kitchen may need some love, too!

The very first thing I recommend you do for your pantry is to invest in good storage. Just as with refrigerated foods, dry foods will have a longer shelf life if they're taken out of their packaging and placed into airtight containers. I like to shop in the bulk bins so I can get exactly the amount I need.

My favorite pantry storage solution are glass mason jars. I use 1-quart (32-ounce) and 2-quart (64-ounce) widemouthed jars. These two sizes allow me to have easily accessible backstock for the most common pantry items and a manageable amount of more sporadically used items.

These are the items I most frequently have stored in my pantry at room temperature:

- Beans (dried and canned)
- Canned items (tomato products, chili, coconut milk, and pumpkin puree)
- Cashews
- Chia seeds
- Cocoa powder
- Dates
- Dried fruits (raisins, apricots, currants)
- Dried mushrooms
- Flaxseeds
- Hemp seeds
- Lentils
- Roasted red peppers (jarred)
- Split peas
- Onions (white, red, and yellow)
- Pecans
- Pine nuts
- Pistachios
- Potatoes (yellow and red) and sweet potatoes
- Pumpkin seeds
- Quinoa
- Sesame seeds
- Shallots
- Sunflower seeds
- Vanilla powder
- Vinegars
- Walnuts
- Whole grains

Because I don't have a traditional built-in pantry space, I've created multiple pantry carts and sections in my fridge, plus storage space for my collection of jars and food storage containers.

FRIDGE-PANTRY CROSSOVER ITEMS

As we've discussed elsewhere in this book, your personal climate and ambient conditions are going to dictate how and where you store your food. Some common dry storage items may benefit from the cooler conditions in your fridge. These include nuts, seeds, different types of flours, and some spices.

Raw Nut and Seed Storage

Raw nuts and seeds will keep for 2 to 3 months in a cool, dry spot in your pantry. But nuts and seeds have high levels of unsaturated fats (that's why we love and need them), so they are inherently delicate. Those fats can turn rancid when exposed to excessive light, heat, and oxygen.

While storing them in containers with tight-fitting lids reduces exposure to oxygen, temperature may still be an issue for you. You can triple the shelf life of your raw nuts and seeds by storing them in the refrigerator. And you can get up to one year of shelf life if they're stored in your freezer. I typically store walnuts, hemp seeds, and ground flaxseeds in my fridge. I like to store them in my crisper drawers or in the door storage. If you live in a humid climate or keep your home on the warm side, you'll want to store raw nuts and seeds closer to your fridge's airflow sources where they'll be kept cooler.

Whole-Grain and Specialty Flours

The very thing that makes whole-grain flours packed with nutrition (the intact bran, germ, and endosperm) also makes them prone to premature spoilage. The bran and germ have natural oils that can go rancid just like the natural oils in nuts and seeds.

Whole-grain flours include:

- Whole wheat
- Oat
- Rye
- Nut and seed flours (like almond flour)
- Bean flours (these don't have as much natural oil)

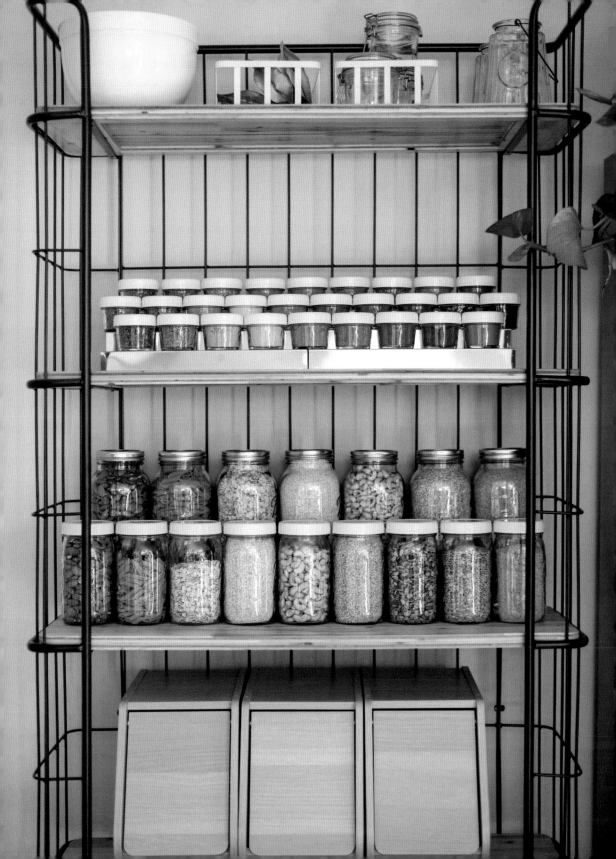

I like to store these flours in my fridge's door storage, but just as I recommended for nuts and seeds, if you live in a humid climate or keep your home warmer, you'll want to store these flours closer to your fridge's airflow sources.

It's also a good idea to quick-freeze the flour in its original packaging before transferring it to a new container and then storing it in the fridge—this will quickly bring down the flour's temperature, which will help maintain optimal cooling temperatures in your fridge.

Whole-grain flours and specialty flours will keep for up to 6 months in the fridge and up to a year in the freezer.

Spices

Many foodies swear by keeping spices in the fridge or freezer to maintain optimal freshness and taste. I don't personally do this, but if you live in a particularly hot and humid environment, this could be helpful. Just be sure that storing spices in the fridge doesn't inadvertently lead to you repeatedly opening the refrigerator door while you're cooking.

Nothing will make you feel more like a real grown-up than taking the time to coordinate your spice storage. It took me thirty-eight years, a pandemic, and the making of this book to get to these pearly gates of adulthood, but let me tell you, it was seriously worth it!

I use mason jars for my spice organization, 4-ounce jars for most and larger 8-ounce jars for the spices I use most frequently, like onion powder, garlic powder, and no-salt seasoning blends. One benefit of using mason jars is that their wider opening makes measuring easier. It's also a convenient storage solution for any spices that come in flat paper or plastic packaging (rather than an airtight bottle).

Generally, you want to store dried herbs and spices in airtight containers with tight-fitting lids and keep them in a cool, dark location in a cupboard, pantry, or drawer. Because I'm constantly developing recipes and move through many of my spices quickly, I'm not so concerned about light exposure, so I keep my spices out in the open, stacked on a three-tier stainless-steel shelf. I see my spice collection as a source of inspiration and beauty that energizes me to get creative in my cooking. There have been many times that I'm sitting at my kitchen table and look over at my pantry cart and get sparked to try out a new flavor combination or recipe.

Your personal approach to spice storage will be dependent on your intention.

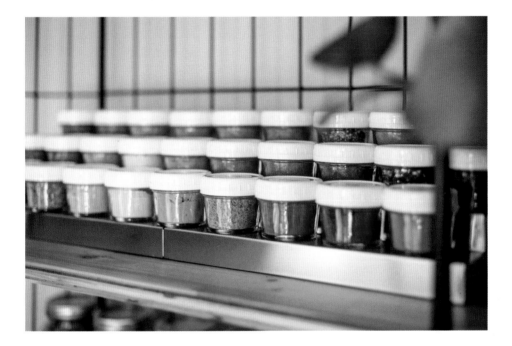

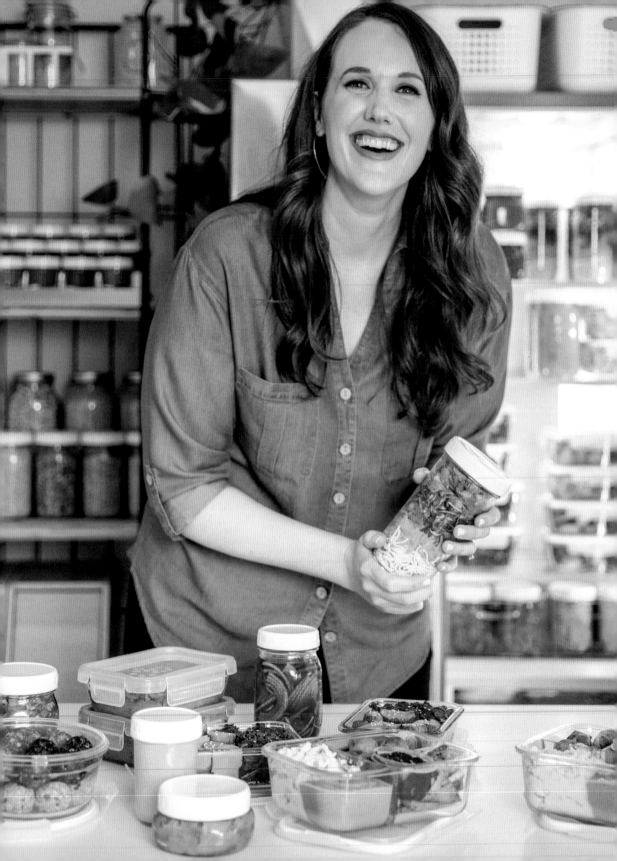

Part 4

RECIPES

These plant-based recipes are simple, adaptable, and delicious, and many have exceptional shelf life in your fridge! The majority of these recipes are quick-to-make, get-you-through-the-week meals. And because I'm a firm believer in putting more produce on your plate, I've packed in as many fruits and veggies as possible. Even if this is your first time eating vegan or plant-based fare, you'll be able to find something you can make and enjoy right now.

The sauces and condiments are designed to help you eat more of the good-for-you stuff without getting in the way of maximizing your nutrition. So instead of loads of oil or sugar, you'll find they're made surprisingly flavorful using whole foods like nuts, fruits, and dates.

Since I'm all about maximizing fridge shelf life, each recipe will have a Storage section that outlines my recommendations for longevity, including specific storage container recommendations. Some recipes will note if the recipe stores well in the freezer. I've found that freezing foods substantially changes the texture to a point where it's no longer appealing to me, so as a general rule I avoid it, except for a few recipes designed to be stored in the freezer.

At the end of most recipes, I'll give you the ways my family and I enjoy eating them. This will usually take the form of simple meal ideas or pointing out when a particular recipe can be used as a component in another recipe.

How the Recipes Are Organized

- **Healthy Fridge Must-Haves (page 167):** These recipes and techniques are the basic ways to ensure you're enjoying more fresh produce from your fridge. They require no cooking and are quick and easy to make.
- **No-Cook Prep (page 174):** I consider these the gold-standard recipes you need to know to get your meal-prep practice off and running—and the best thing is, there's absolutely no cooking required! If you're interested in reaping the benefits of weekly batch cooking but you don't want to make things overly complicated, these are the recipes to start with.
- **Cooked Prep (page 226):** Layer these recipes onto your no-cook preps when you're ready to level up to weekly meal prepping. These are quick-cooking, fresh, and flavorful recipes that keep for at least 9 days in the fridge.
- **Scratch-Made Extras (page 304):** These are simple DIY recipes for some everyday items like veggie broths and plant milks, as well as a few sweets with ingredients that you can mostly source from bulk bins.
- **On-Demand Favorites (page 317):** These are recipes you can make at a moment's notice using recipe components you already have prepped like

sauces, dressings, or plant proteins. They can help you get a variety of meals from your weekly prepping practice and taste best when they're made to order.

Remember how I asked you to identify your fridge goals at the beginning of the book (page 12)? Here's the breakdown of how these recipe categories align with your goals:

- **GOAL:** The Fresh Fridge → **RECIPES:** Healthy Fridge Must-Haves
- **GOAL:** The Chopped Fridge → **RECIPES:** Healthy Fridge Must-Haves, In-Fridge Salad Bar (page 174), Salad Jar Preps (page 293), Fridge Pickles (page 198); chop and store the components for the No-Cook Prep and Cooked Prep recipes
- **GOAL:** The No-Cook Fridge → **RECIPES:** No-Cook Prep plus anything from the Chopped Fridge above
- **GOAL:** The Prepped Fridge → **RECIPES:** No-Cook Prep, Cooked Prep, and On-Demand Favorites
- **GOAL:** The Ecofriendly Fridge → **RECIPES:** Scratch-Made Extras and then pick your level of processing above

Equipment

I'm a big fan of the basics, and I don't like having a ton of kitchen gadgets. But there are some items I do recommend, so I've listed those for you here. A few are essential, and a few are nice to have but not required.
- **Whisk:** For the smoothest mixed sauces.
- **High-speed blender:** I'm specifically talking about a Vitamix- or Blendtec-caliber blender. I know I'm not supposed to play favorites, but these machines seem to be the most consistent when breaking down nuts, dates, and frozen fruit; a standard blender may not be powerful enough to smoothly blend these ingredients.

A Note about Blender Jars: Another factor to consider is the size of the blender jar (the vessel that holds the food to be blended). Some of the recipes intentionally yield smaller amounts so you can experiment with flavors and techniques that might be new to you. If your blender jar is wider than 4 inches, you may have trouble blending some of these smaller-yield recipes, so please be mindful.

- **Food processor:** I only consider this an essential item if you plan on making any of the Fridge Bite recipes on pages 222–225 or the Plant-Based Protein recipes on pages 270–279. If you have one, you can use the slicing and shredding blades to prep your weekly salad bar toppings.

- **Cookie scoop:** This is a really helpful tool for healthy eating because it gives you a precision measurement (I like the 1-ounce/2-tablespoon size) and releases the food easily. This can help you portion prepped foods quickly and efficiently.

- **Garlic press:** Garlic adds tremendous flavor to your cooking; a garlic press saves serious time when you need finely minced garlic.

- **Canning funnel:** This is another prepping-specific item I love having on hand. It helps you quickly and cleanly transfer sauces, soups, and cooked foods into glass jars. I have both a regular-mouth plastic funnel and a widemouthed stainless-steel funnel.

- **Mini measuring spoons:** While a standard measuring spoon set only goes down to ¼ teaspoon, this set includes spoons for smaller increments, usually tad, dash, pinch, smidgen, and drop. These run about $6 on Amazon and are wonderful for precise seasoning. However, aside from the occasional pinch and dash, I don't use any of the other sizes in the recipes in this book, so these aren't essential.

- **Multiple sets of dry measuring cups and spoons:** Having to rinse things out as I batch cook slows me down, so I have a collection of cheap dry measuring cups and spoons that I keep in a basket in my cupboard. You can find measuring cup sets for as little as a dollar or two; I've even thrifted a few of mine.

Ingredients

Here's a quick rundown of some of my most often used ingredients, as well as some specialty ingredients you'll see in the recipes. These are some of my secret weapons in the flavor department!

FREQUENTLY USED INGREDIENTS

- **Tahini sauce:** This is a staple condiment in Middle Eastern and Mediterranean cuisine with a nutty, earthy flavor and creamy texture. It's made from ground hulled sesame seeds and is naturally vegan and gluten-free. I love using this as an oil replacement in dressings and sauces because it has more phytonutrients and intact fiber than oil, while still providing fat and richness. I like to keep tahini in my spice cabinet to preserve its runny consistency. I do go through tahini quickly, using up opened jars within a few weeks.

- **No-salt seasoning:** These are spice blends with no added salt or sugar. My favorite no-salt seasoning for cooking is Costco's Kirkland brand organic no-salt seasoning. I like using Sprouts Farmers Market brand organic salt-free garlic and herb seasoning as a kind of "finishing salt," which is just a fancy way of saying that I love sprinkling it on top of my salads and soups.

- **Roasted red peppers:** These are a pantry staple in my home, and I love using them in recipes to add a sweet, slightly spicy flavor and amazing color. Look for jarred roasted red peppers that don't have added oil.

- **Canned light or reduced-fat coconut milk:** This is another pantry staple that I like to have on hand and is featured in several recipes. The difference between coconut cream, regular coconut milk, and light coconut milk is the ratio of water to fat they contain; coconut cream contains the most fat, and light coconut milk the most water. No matter what type you use, always shake the can or stir before using, as the creamiest parts will cling to the top of the can. You can substitute regular coconut milk for light—just note that it's much thicker and will change the consistency of the dish as a result. If you've opened a can of coconut milk but don't end up using it all, empty the rest into a glass jar with a tight-fitting lid and store on an upper fridge shelf toward the back or close to an airflow source. It will stay good for up to 2 weeks.

- **Vegetable broth:** Vegetable broth is a great substitute for oil when cooking and sautéing, and you'll find it used in many of my recipes. I like using it to deglaze the pan when I'm sautéing veggies or adjust the consistency of sauces. And of course you'll see it used as a base for soup. I've included an easy recipe for veggie broth on page 314.
- **Almond milk:** This is my personal favorite type of plant milk, but when you see it called for in a recipe, feel free to substitute your own favorite type. I've included a recipe for almond milk that can be made sweet or unsweetened on page 304.
- **Medjool dates:** One of the most important steps I took in my health journey was learning to live without sugar. Instead of relying on sugar to sweeten recipes, I use dates. They naturally contain a fruit sugar called fructose and have a sweet, caramel-like taste. Look for fresh, plump Medjool dates; when they look more shriveled, it means they are drier and not as fresh, which can make them harder to blend or break down during cooking. I store dates in my cupboard in a glass jar with a tight-fitting lid; keeping them at room temperature maintains their softer texture.
- **Maple syrup:** This is another great sweetener and more accessible than dates for many people.
- **Firm tofu:** I use tofu a lot, especially in the Plant-Based Protein recipes on pages 270–279. I buy my tofu in bulk, where it typically comes in 16-ounce blocks, but 14-ounce packages are what you're most likely to find in stores; you can use either weight for the recipes in this book.

SPECIALTY INGREDIENTS

- **Nutritional yeast:** These crispy flakes provide an umami flavor that mimics the flavor profiles of eggs and dairy. Nutritional yeast can be found in the spice aisle of most grocery stores.
- **White (light) miso paste:** This is a Japanese condiment made from fermented soybeans. It provides a distinctive salty and umami flavor with less sodium than other salt substitutes. My preferred brand is Miso Master's organic mellow white miso. Miso is typically found in the refrigerated section of the grocery. Do not substitute darker miso pastes, as the taste will be much stronger. I store miso in my deli drawer or inner fridge door storage (closest to the door hinges), and it keeps for many months.

- **Vanilla powder:** This black powder is simply ground dried vanilla beans. It gives you amazing vanilla flavor without the alcohol aftertaste you typically get with vanilla extract. My preferred manufacturer is Wilderness Poets, and they ship throughout the US. Of all the specialty ingredients I recommend, this one is the most expensive and difficult to find. While I firmly believe this ingredient makes a big difference in the sweet recipes in this book, you can substitute an equal quantity of vanilla extract or use seeds scraped from a vanilla bean (I'll indicate how many vanilla beans in the recipe). I store opened containers of vanilla powder in my fridge in the door storage area or in a drawer.
- **Reduced-sodium tamari:** While soy sauce is made with both soy and wheat, tamari is made entirely (or almost entirely) from soy, with no (or little) wheat. (Not all tamari is gluten-free; if you avoid gluten, be sure to check the label.) Tamari has a richer, deeper flavor than soy sauce. You can substitute soy sauce if that's what you have on hand, just note that the flavor will be a bit different and you'll need to adjust the amount to account for the sodium content. I store this condiment in the door storage area of my fridge.
- **Liquid aminos and coconut aminos:** Both liquid aminos and coconut aminos are good substitutes for soy sauce. Liquid aminos are made from treating soybeans with an acidic solution to break them down into free amino acids. They add a savory, salty flavor and are gluten-free (whereas soy sauce is traditionally made with wheat). Tamari is a good substitute if you can't find liquid aminos. I store this condiment in my spice cabinet. Coconut aminos are made from fermented coconut blossom nectar with a little bit of added salt. They are soy-free and have a sweeter taste than liquid aminos. I store this condiment in the door storage area of my fridge. I wouldn't recommend substituting coconut aminos for liquid aminos or vice versa, as the flavors are different.
- **Liquid smoke:** I've included this condiment in a couple of the Plant-Based Protein recipes. It helps reproduce a meaty flavor that some people enjoy, especially if they're omnivores or new to vegan eating. My meat-eating hubby really enjoys dishes that incorporate this flavoring. Just keep in mind that a little bit of this goes a very long way and some people can find it overpowering. I store this condiment in my spice cabinet.

- **Bean pasta:** I can't express how much I love bean pasta! Probably the greatest health invention of the past decade, it blesses you with the manifold benefits of whole legumes, and making the switch to bean pasta will naturally help you with pasta portion control and aid in your insulin response to high-glycemic foods. Bean pasta can take some getting used to, as it has a heartier texture, more robust bean flavor, and higher fiber content than conventional pastas. Look for bean pastas with only one to three listed ingredients, and always try to cook the pasta to slightly al dente—this gives the cooked pasta a longer shelf life in the fridge and prevents it from breaking down when mixed with sauces.

How to Start Meal Prepping

I've been consistently prepping for over four years now, and it's made all the difference in converting sporadic healthy eating into a true lifestyle.

If you're new to meal prepping, the recipes in this book will provide you with plenty of easy, healthy options. But here is my advice to you: Batch cooking can be intimidating—don't fall into the trap of trying to change your whole life in one week. Instead, try the following steps for a natural and sustainable progression into weekly meal prepping.

1. **Where should you start? Breakfast.** It's easy and manageable, and since breakfast time is usually when things are the most hectic and rushed anyway, why not have something ready to go? Start with choosing a recipe from one of these recipe categories:
   - Smoothie Freezer Packs (pages 203–208)
   - Overnight Oats (pages 209–213)
   - Chia Pudding (pages 217–221)
2. **No-cook lunches:** Once you get consistent at breakfast preps, try branching out to lunch. Pick no-cook recipes from these sections:
   - In-Fridge Salad Bar Basics (pages 174–181)
   - Plant-Powered Mayo Salads (pages 214–216)
   - Greek Salad Jars (page 294)
   - Rainbow Salad Jars (page 295)

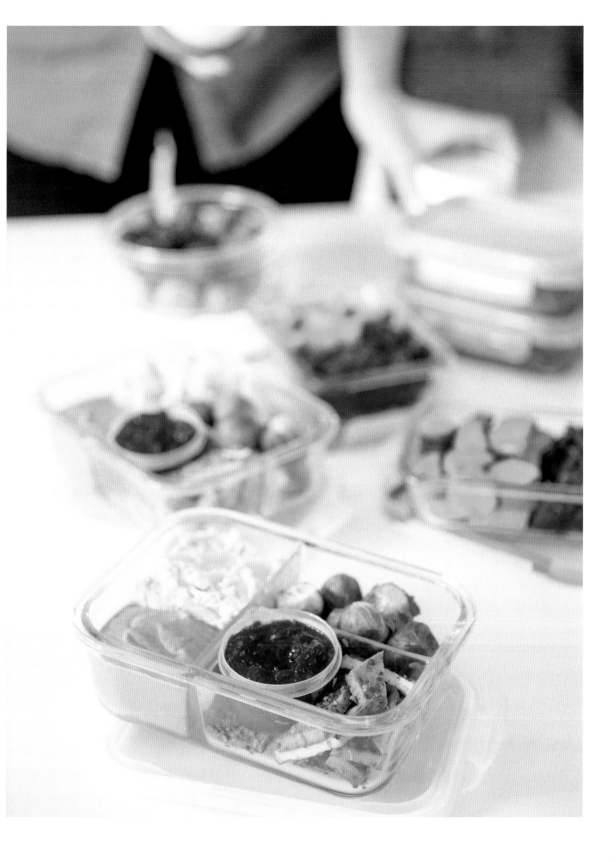

3. **Cooked lunches and dinners:** The next step is to move on to doing cooked preps for dinners and lunches. The Cooked Prepping recipes (pages 226–239) are designed for weekly batch-prepping. But if this is your very first time batch cooking, I actually suggest that you *begin your prepping practice with recipes you already know and love* rather than attempting brand-new ones. Peruse the recipes in that section for ideas and see what similar recipes you already know that could work for the week (or, realistically, part of the week). A batch of your favorite soup is perfect to start; then select two or three more of your favorite recipes that you know will keep in the fridge for at least 4 to 5 days. Add an In-Fridge Salad Bar (pages 174–181) and one or two Quick-Mix Sauces (pages 168–173) to round things out. Follow this formula for at least 2 weeks.

4. **Add something new:** For the third week, try switching in a new recipe—for example, one of the healthy, flavorful soups on pages 226–239.

5. **Keep going:** For week 4, after three solid weeks of batch cooking, try incorporating two new recipes. For example, add one selection from the One-Pot Meals and Sides category (pages 259–268) and one from the 4-Step Preps category (pages 280–292).

Each of us has a different body with different nutrition needs and appetite levels. The only way to learn how much you need to prep is by trying it out and learning what works for you! By the end of your first month of prepping, you'll have a realistic idea of how much you actually eat and how much you need to prep. Now that you know what works best for you, explore all the recipes in this book to find new favorites!

Making These Recipes Work for Everyone

All the recipes in this book are plant-based and made from whole foods. But since I'm the only vegan in my family—my husband and kids eat and enjoy a ton of plant-based foods but also eat meat and dairy—I've made it very easy to add meat and dairy to the recipes I'm sharing with you here.

Let me give you a few examples: My hubby loves Crunchy Thai Noodle Salad Jars (page 300), and I often prep them for both of us for the week. For myself, I make a batch of Easy Baked Tofu (page 271), and for him, I prep cooked chicken strips to add to his salads. My son adds dairy sour cream and cheese to his bowls of Oil-Free Fire-Roasted Smoky Chili (page 265). My daughter loves Un-Fried Rice (page 259), but likes me to add scrambled eggs to her portion.

All these dishes are customizable and can be made to accommodate animal products. What we can all feel good about is that at the heart of these recipes, there are whole foods and loads of veggies.

The Nutritarian Lifestyle

A Nutritarian is a person who habitually eats a high-nutrient, whole-food, plant-based diet; avoids processed foods; and cooks without oil and excess salt. The term was coined by Dr. Joel Furhman with the intention of getting people to think about and concentrate on the protective nutrients in foods instead of just the calories, protein, carbs, and fat.

Nutritarians strive for health excellence, basing food decisions on how health-protective and lifespan-increasing a food is. Many turn to this lifestyle to reverse or prevent food-related illnesses, cancers, and immune system conditions. I came into this lifestyle to help me recover from lifelong food addiction, binge eating, and obesity.

On the surface, the Nutritarian lifestyle can seem very restrictive, but that's mainly because of the prevalence of the Standard American Diet (low intake of fresh produce, emphasis on meat and dairy) and our modern profit-driven food landscape.

While this book is for all kinds of eaters, I want to share the guiding Nutritarian principles that have had the biggest impact on my health:

- **Emphasize micronutrients:** Nutritarians make their food choices based on which foods have the highest concentrations of micronutrients. Micronutrients are the vitamins, minerals, fiber, and phytochemicals found in natural plant foods. Phytochemicals (also called phytonutrients) are complex chemical compounds that occur naturally in plants. They work synergistically together within your body to maximize your genetic potential by sweeping out toxins, reducing inflammation, protecting blood vessels, repairing cellular and DNA damage, inhibiting fat storage, and protecting you from cancer and chronic disease. Thousands of these compounds have been identified, and thousands more have yet to be discovered. Nutritarians try to get as wide a variety of phytochemicals into their diet as possible and understand that our bodies actually "crave" these phytonutrients for proper functioning.

- **Eat more veggies:** Nutritarians aim to eat 1 pound of cooked veggies and 1 pound of raw veggies daily. I know this seems like a shocking amount of veggies, because it's considerably more than is typical for the Standard American Diet. Raw and cooked veggies are given equal priority because certain nutrients and enzymes are degraded during cooking, while others are enhanced. By making it a priority to eat both, you're ensuring the most benefit for your body. Raw foods have high fiber and water content, so they keep you feeling full longer and with fewer calories than their cooked counterparts (cooking condenses the natural sugars in vegetables and concentrates their calories).

- **Make fruits and dates your go-to sweeteners:** Nutritarians eat fresh fruit for dessert for the majority of meals and enjoy fruit- and date-sweetened treats a few times a week. Humans have an inherent "sweet tooth," but we're meant to crave fructose, the natural sugar found in fruit and dates. These retain their natural fiber (which helps to properly regulate insulin response) and phytochemicals.

- **Replace oil with whole, intact fats:** Oil is a processed food. The natural fat is stripped from its fiber, which concentrates the calories and makes them easier (too easy, in fact) for our body to absorb into the bloodstream, because there's nothing our body needs to break down or process for itself. While fat is hugely important for the proper absorption of nutrients, you want to get yours from whole, intact sources. It's healthier to eat actual olives than their oil. Nutritarians replace oil with raw nuts and seeds and avocado.

- **Limit sodium:** Excessive salt and sodium intake deadens your taste buds (making it harder to enjoy the more subtle flavors of natural foods), contributes to compulsive overeating, and causes chronic health problems, including high blood pressure, heart attack, stroke, and certain types of cancer. Nutritarians strive to consume no more than 1,000 milligrams of sodium daily. A natural, unprocessed, plant-based diet provides 500 to 700 milligrams of sodium daily, so Nutritarians try not to add more than 300 to 500 milligrams of sodium.

Healthy Fridge Must-Haves

I designed these recipes and techniques to be the perfect starting place for developing your fresh fridge practice. All you need to make these recipes happen are a knife, a whisk, a mixing bowl, and a few storage jars.

PRODUCE SNACK JARS

Nothing will ensure that you grab a healthy, fresh snack more than having these easy-to-make jars lined up smartly in your fridge. This is my way of luring readers who are interested in eating fresh produce into the very beginning steps of meal prepping. We're talking as easy as it could possibly get, with no cooking and the use of store-bought components. These jars have become a mainstay in our work-and-school-from-home quarantine lives, as they're infinitely customizable and self-serve for the kids!

EASY VEGGIE CUPS

Carrots, celery, bell peppers, and/or radishes
Store-bought hummus and/or guacamole cups (see Note)

Cut carrots, celery, and bell peppers into 3¼-inch sticks. Radishes can be left whole or halved. You can do a blend of the veggies or one type in each jar. My kids like carrots and celery.

Place the veggies in widemouthed 1-pint jar(s) and add 1 inch to 1½ inches of cool water (do not add water to jars with bell peppers). Place the hummus or guacamole cup in the jar on top of the veggies and seal the lid of the jar.

Storage: Cups without bell peppers will keep for 9 to 12 days in the fridge. Cups with bell pepper sticks sliced 1 inch wide will keep for 7 to 9 days; cups with thinner bell pepper sticks will keep for 5 to 7 days.

Note: Look for 2- to 2.5-ounce cups no more than 3 inches in diameter; I use Kirkland brand hummus and Good Foods guacamole. You could also use homemade hummus and/or guacamole; store them in small plastic sauce containers, either inside the jars or separately, depending on the size of your containers.

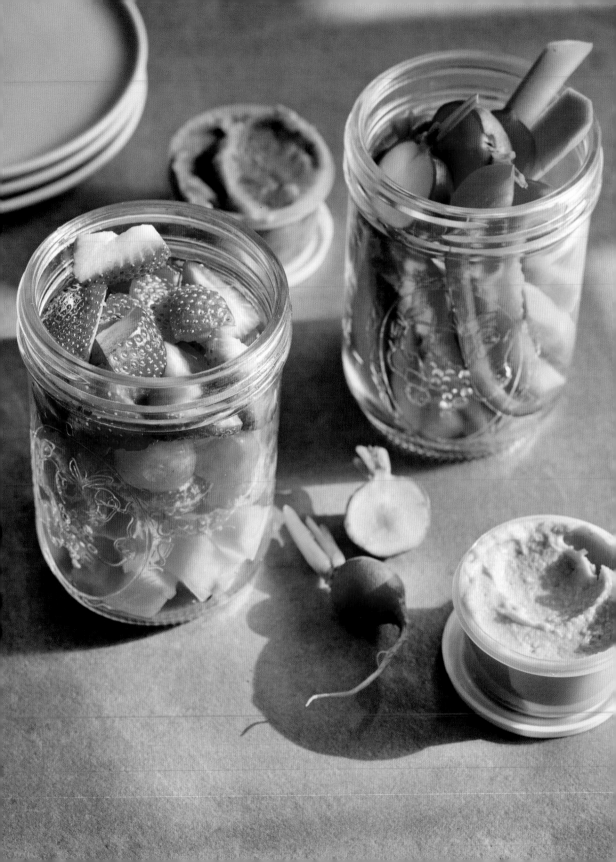

EASY FRUIT CUPS

Strawberries

Mandarin oranges

Kiwifruit (optional)

Fresh pineapple chunks

Grapes

Wash the strawberries, then hull and quarter them. Peel and segment the mandarins. Peel and chop the kiwi (if using). Place the fruit in 1-pint glass jar(s), then seal the lids.

For simple layered "sunset" cups, start with pineapple, add mandarin segments, and top with strawberries.

For rainbow fruit cups, layer red grapes on the bottom, then kiwi, pineapple, and mandarins, and top with strawberries.

Storage: Cups made without kiwi will keep for 7 to 9 days in the fridge. Cups with kiwi keep for 4 to 5 days (especially if you keep the kiwi chunks larger), but they get the kids feeling excited (because, hello, rainbows!) and have always been a favorite on social media. Note that strawberries may dry out a bit during storage but will still taste good.

Note: Mandarin oranges, pineapple, and grapes have the longest shelf life (7 to 9 days). Kiwis have a shorter shelf life (4 to 5 days), and the strawberries' texture will change slightly during storage. Take these factors into consideration when choosing which fruits to use.

QUICK-MIX SAUCES

Making homemade sauces and dressings was one of the simplest changes I made when I first started out with healthy eating. This small area of change also had an instant impact on my health. I got to control how much salt, sweetness, or viscosity I needed to feel satisfied, and it was always considerably less than store-bought. I've curated this collection of five amazingly tasty oil-free sauces and dressings to serve as your introduction to going homemade. The yields are smaller so you can experiment and find your favorites; once you do, it's easy to make a double batch.

Notes:

- These sauces use tahini or nut/seed butter in place of oil. Because these are mixable sauces, you want to make sure that your tahini or nut/seed butter is runny and well incorporated, or the final result may be lumpy. Using the pasty, mostly solid tahini at the bottom of the jar will give you poor results.
- These sauces will thicken after their first night in the fridge. To thin them, I recommend stirring in no more than 2 teaspoons of water at a time and mixing well until your desired consistency is reached.

Clockwise from top right: Golden Turmeric Sauce (page 173), Lemon-Garlic Tahini Sauce (page 172), Peanut Coconut Sauce (opposite), Creamy Balsamic Dressing (opposite), and Tahini Yum Sauce (page 172)

PEANUT COCONUT SAUCE

MAKES 1¾ CUPS (SEVEN ¼-CUP SERVINGS)

½ cup canned reduced-fat coconut milk
½ tablespoon maple syrup
½ cup salted peanut butter
¼ cup water
1½ tablespoons coconut aminos

In a small bowl, whisk together the coconut milk, maple syrup, peanut butter, water, and coconut aminos until well combined.

Storage: Store in the fridge in a glass food storage container or ½-pint glass jar with a tight-fitting lid for 9 to 12 days.

Enjoy!

This creamy, savory sauce is used for dipping Rainbow Collard Wraps (page 322) and as a salad dressing for Crunchy Thai Noodle Salad Jars (page 300). I personally love it drizzled on Sweet Potato and Kale Prep Bowls (page 283), or tossed with warm pasta and bell peppers and garnished with chopped roasted peanuts and fresh cilantro. Some of the recipe testers who helped on this book loved it with an added squeeze of lime juice or sriracha! Other testers enjoyed it as a simmer sauce for chicken and veggies.

CREAMY BALSAMIC DRESSING

MAKES 1 CUP (FOUR ¼-CUP SERVINGS)

⅓ cup tahini
⅓ cup balsamic vinegar
¼ cup water
1 tablespoon maple syrup
½ teaspoon Dijon mustard

In a small bowl, whisk together the tahini, vinegar, and water. Add the maple syrup and mustard and stir until well mixed.

Storage: Store in the fridge in a glass food storage container or ½-pint glass jar with a tight-fitting lid for up to 14 days.

Enjoy!

Some recipe testers preferred adding double the Dijon! This sweet-and-tangy dressing is my recommended beginner dressing for your In-Fridge Salad Bar (page 174).

A few of my favorite salad combinations for this dressing:
- Kale, sliced apple, and pepitas
- Chopped raw broccoli, chopped kale, chopped apple, grated carrots, minced red onions, and raisins or dried currants

TAHINI YUM SAUCE

MAKES 1 CUP (FOUR ¼-CUP SERVINGS)

½ cup tahini
½ cup water
1 tablespoon coconut aminos
2 teaspoons Dijon mustard
1½ teaspoons no-salt seasoning (see page 159)

In a small bowl, whisk together the tahini and water. Add the coconut aminos, mustard, and seasoning and stir until well mixed.

Storage: Store in the fridge in a glass food storage container or ½-pint glass jar with a tight-fitting lid for up to 14 days.

Enjoy!

This has become my go-to veggie-roasting sauce and is a more nutritious alternative to olive oil. Simply toss with your favorite vegetables, sprinkle with a little salt, if desired, and roast. I also use this sauce as a salad dressing that even my eight-year-old likes!

LEMON-GARLIC TAHINI SAUCE

MAKES ABOUT 1 CUP (ABOUT FOUR ¼-CUP SERVINGS)

⅓ cup plus 1 tablespoon tahini
⅓ cup plus 1 tablespoon water
3 tablespoons plus 1 teaspoon lemon juice
2 large garlic cloves, minced or pressed
2 tablespoons chopped fresh dill, or 2 teaspoons dried (see Note)
Salt and ground black pepper

In a small bowl, whisk together the tahini and water. Add the lemon juice, garlic, and dill. Season with salt and pepper and stir until well mixed.

Storage: Store in the fridge in a glass food storage container or ½-pint glass jar with a tight-fitting lid for up to 14 days.

Enjoy!

My hubby and I can't get enough of this sauce, which seems to go with absolutely everything we throw at it. I use it as a sauce for Falafel Prep Bowls (page 288), and it's also amazing drizzled over a baked potato, tossed with warm pasta, as a salad dressing, or as a dipping sauce for warm pita bread and crudités.

Note: I love this sauce with extra dill—you can add as much as you like!

GOLDEN TURMERIC SAUCE

MAKES ABOUT ¾ CUP (THREE ¼-CUP SERVINGS)

⅓ cup tahini
⅓ cup water
2 tablespoons lemon or lime juice
1 large garlic clove, minced or pressed
1 teaspoon minced or grated fresh ginger
¼ teaspoon salt
¼ teaspoon curry powder
¼ to ½ teaspoon ground turmeric

In a small bowl, whisk together the tahini, water, and lemon juice. Add the garlic, ginger, salt, curry powder, and turmeric and stir until well mixed.

Storage: Store in the fridge in a glass food storage container or ½-pint glass jar with a tight-fitting lid for up to 9 days.

Enjoy!

This is my preferred sauce for Sweet Potato and Kale Prep Bowls (page 283). I'll often use it as a salad dressing or for roasting veggies (onions, bell peppers, and carrots work beautifully). This is also an amazing sauce to add to boiled potatoes for a healthier potato salad—I like to stir in red bell pepper and fresh cilantro, too.

Note: If you're new to plant-based eating, I recommend starting with one of the other tahini-based sauces first. Some of our recipe testers liked to add a bit of maple syrup to balance out the flavor. This may help you if you find the combination of tahini and turmeric to be bitter-tasting.

No-Cook Prep Recipes

Now we're getting into the heart of what this book is all about: making your fridge the most powerful tool for your health. I want you to open your fridge doors and be greeted by a rainbow of colorful, ready-to-eat produce, meals, snacks, and healthful options to fuel a busy and vibrant life!

I like to think of these recipes as your "first prep in the right direction," as they don't require a lot of time and involve no cooking. In fact, at certain times of year, turning on my stove or oven is just about the last thing in the world I want to do. Enter this collection of recipes that require no heating whatsoever!

IN-FRIDGE SALAD BAR BASICS

Probably the biggest reason I've been able to stay so consistent at my healthy lifestyle has been understanding the power of eating salad regularly. In fact, if there's only one change you're willing to make in your diet, let it be this: eating a large salad as your "main dish" for at least one meal a day. It's the most basic and powerful nutritarian tenet and helped me release over 80 pounds.

After chronically binge eating for most of my adult life, filling myself up with nutrient- and fiber-rich salads helped curb my desire to overeat processed foods, while providing my body with the real nutrients it needs. Today, if I don't get in at least one large salad each day, I can immediately notice a difference in my energy levels.

While there are a couple of ways to prep salads for the week, an in-fridge salad bar is my favorite way to go because it's so versatile. I can bring out all our prepped greens and toppings and have the kids create their own customized salads for dinner. Or I can also use the chopped salad bar ingredients in other recipes (I also have six "salad jar" recipes for you later in the book, starting on page 293).

When planning your in-fridge salad bar, the most important thing to figure out is how much to prep. That will depend on these factors:

- How big will each salad be?
- How many people are you prepping for?
- How long do you want the salad bar to last?

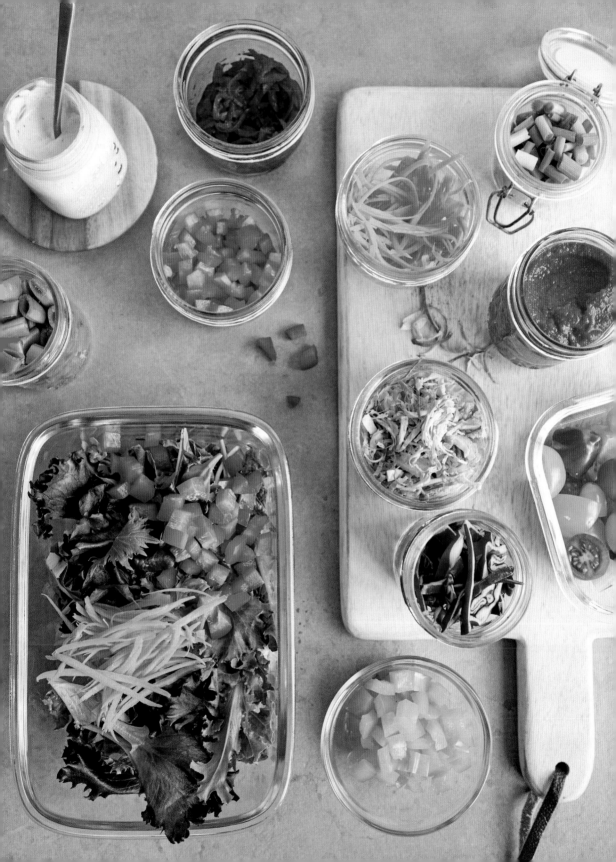

Salad Size

Decide how big you want to make your salads and how many salads you want to make for the week, then chop and prep the ingredients accordingly. There was definitely a bit of a learning curve when I first started my large-salad-a-day habit. Salads should be *big*—that means they should have at least 1½ to 2 cups (packed) of greens or lettuce and ¾ to 1 cup of fresh, crunchy toppings. If you don't usually eat a lot of salads, you may want to start with a smaller serving and work up. But I promise that if you eat large salads consistently, you'll notice a big difference in your energy levels.

Prepping for the Family

If you're prepping for your partner and/or kids, decide what size salads they're likely to eat. Next, decide how often you think they will have a salad. Type this up on your computer or phone (remember to include your information, too!) so you can easily plan your weekly salad bars in the future. If certain family members prefer certain toppings to others, create your salad bar accordingly.

Storage

I like to prep enough salad fixings to last us at least 7 days. Some weeks I can only manage a mini prep session, and the salad bar lasts for more like 4 to 5 days. Decide on a time frame that feels most comfortable to you. The overall duration of your salad bar is dependent on the shelf life of its individual components. (See the produce storage guide starting on page 88 for more information.) When I have a topping that I know has a shorter shelf life, I consciously go heavy on that topping for my salads in the beginning of the week and reserve the longer-lasting toppings for the end of the week.

I've found that glass containers work best to maintain the temperature of salad bar components, since you'll have to have them out on the counter or table while you and your family make their salads. I like to use glass snap-lock food storage containers or glass jars. For glass jars, I recommend using plastic lids instead of two-piece metal; they are easier to open and close and more convenient for frequent use. I also corral all the containers for my in-fridge salad bar in a large plastic bin so it's easy to pull everything out.

SALAD BAR PLANNING GUIDE

Choose 1 or 2 types of lettuce/greens:

Baby mixed greens

Baby spinach

Butter lettuce

Iceberg lettuce

Leaf lettuce

Curly kale

Romaine

Choose 3 or 4 rainbow veggies:

Beets, shredded raw, pickled, or roasted

Bell peppers (orange, red, yellow)

Cabbage (red, green), shredded raw or pickled

Carrots

Cauliflower

Celery

Cucumbers

Radishes: raw or pickled

Tomatoes (cherry and grape store best in the fridge)

Onion (green, red, yellow, white), raw or pickled

BONUS! Choose 1 powerhouse green veggie:

Broccoli

Brussels sprouts, shaved raw

Microgreens (kale, broccoli, radish)

Sugar snap peas

Add optional healthy toppings:

Avocado (try to pair this topping with an oil-free dressing)

Beans (cooked or canned)

Fresh fruits (apples, berries, citrus, mangoes, pears, pineapple, pomegranates)

Dried fruits (raisins, currants, chopped apricots)

Raw nuts and seeds

Salt-free seasonings

Fresh herbs, chopped

Colorful fingerling potatoes (the more color, the more nutrients), steamed

Must-Know Cooked Veggies (pages 246–252)

Fridge Pickles (pages 198–202)

Choose 1 or 2 dressings:

Quick-Mix Sauces (pages 168–173)

Blended dressings (pages 195–197)

Savory hummus (pages 183–185)

Vinegar

Citrus juice

A Note about Dressings

You don't want to get in the way of a good thing by drowning all those nutrient-rich fresh greens and veggies with loads of hard-to-process, calorie-dense dressing. Most of the dressing recipes in this book contain no refined oil, and all are delicious. But depending on your lifestyle, you may prefer a store-bought dressing or homemade vinaigrette. If you're trying to maximize your health, I recommend avoiding creamy dairy-based dressings. Be mindful of how much you're using, with the ultimate goal of using less and enjoying the natural flavor of the produce more.

SIMPLE RAINBOW HUMMUS SALAD

My number one goal when creating a salad is to get in the widest variety of nutrients I can, and a fun way to do that is by matching my salad toppings to the rainbow! This is the basic, get-you-started rainbow salad because the toppings are easy to find and have an overall long shelf life. It's the salad I eat most frequently, followed by cooked soup or a prep bowl, for lunch.

MAKES 1 SERVING

1½ to 2 cups chopped leaf lettuce
¼ to ½ cup halved grape tomatoes
¼ to ½ cup chopped cucumber
2 tablespoons to ¼ cup shredded carrot
2 tablespoons to ¼ cup chopped yellow bell pepper
2 tablespoons to ¼ cup diced green onions or pickled red onion (see page 198)
2 tablespoons to ¼ cup chopped red cabbage
¼ to ⅓ cup Classic Hummus (page 183)
Balsamic vinegar or pickling liquid
Raw or toasted sesame seeds or no-salt seasoning (see page 159), for garnish (optional)

Arrange the lettuce in a large bowl and top with the tomatoes, cucumber, carrot, bell pepper, onion, and cabbage. Top with the hummus and drizzle with vinegar. Garnish with sesame seeds, if desired, and enjoy.

Note: You could also use your favorite store-bought hummus or vinaigrette.

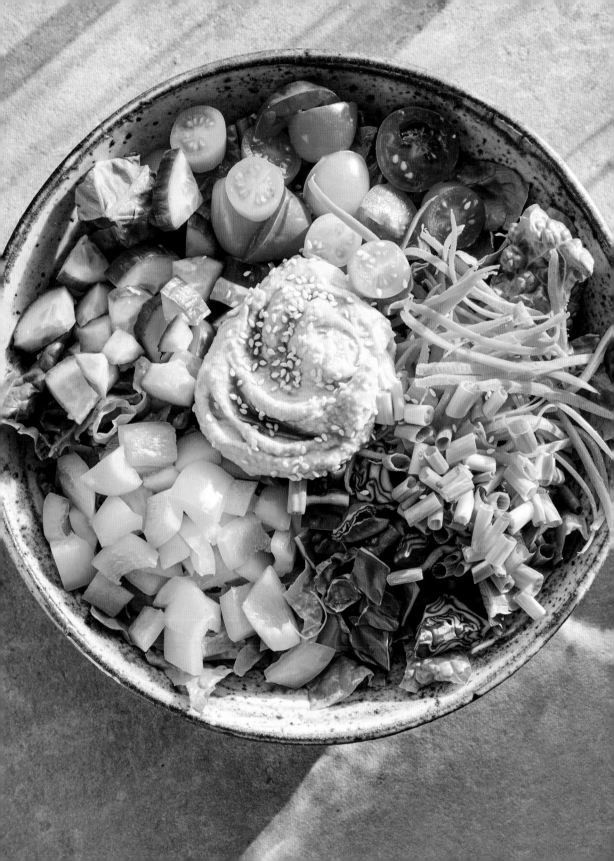

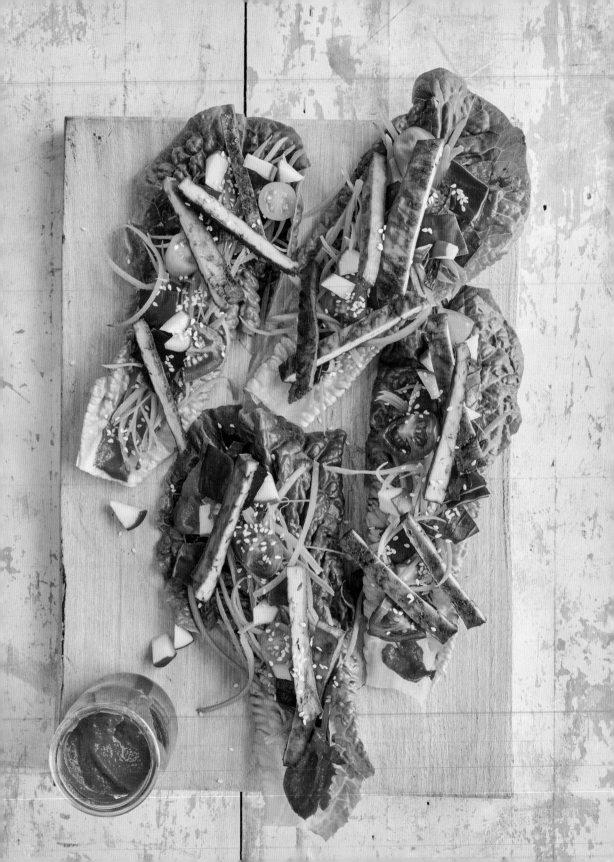

COLORFUL LETTUCE BOATS

Sometimes presenting the same ingredients in a unique way is all it takes for a meal to feel special and different. I like making these lettuce boats in lieu of a salad when I need some extra self-pampering, because they're so beautiful to look at and have an amazing combination of flavors and textures!

MAKES 1 SERVING

6 tablespoons Classic Hummus (page 183) or Beet Hummus (page 184)

4 or 5 romaine lettuce leaves

3 or 4 grape tomatoes, halved

¼ cup chopped red cabbage

¼ cup chopped radishes

2 tablespoons shredded carrot

Sesame seeds (optional)

3 or 4 strips Easy Baked Tofu (page 271; optional, if you want to make these more of a full meal)

Spread 1 to 2 tablespoons of the hummus onto each romaine leaf. Top with the tomatoes, cabbage, radishes, and carrot. Sprinkle with sesame seeds and top with the tofu, if desired, then enjoy.

Note: You can use your favorite store-bought hummus. For extra flavor, you could also add a dipping sauce like Peanut Coconut Sauce (page 171).

OIL-FREE HUMMUS

You can make delicious homemade hummus without added oil. Beans are absolutely amazing for your health, so it's a great idea to eat them daily; these sweet and savory hummus recipes are creamy and decadent-tasting and a great way to eat all the fresh fruit and veggies!

The size and power of your blender matters a lot when making smooth and creamy homemade hummus. Be mindful of the bottom width of your blender jar. For hummus recipes that yield less than 3 cups, it's best to use a blender jar with a base no wider than 4 inches, or use a smaller attachment (if using a Vitamix Ascent series blender).

Storage: These hummus recipes will keep for at least 10 days when stored in a glass food storage container or glass jar with a tight-fitting lid.

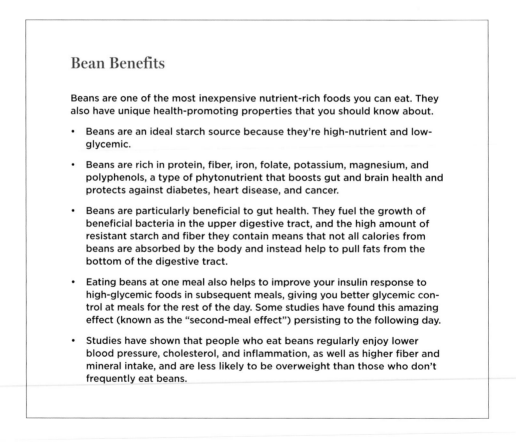

Bean Benefits

Beans are one of the most inexpensive nutrient-rich foods you can eat. They also have unique health-promoting properties that you should know about.

- Beans are an ideal starch source because they're high-nutrient and low-glycemic.

- Beans are rich in protein, fiber, iron, folate, potassium, magnesium, and polyphenols, a type of phytonutrient that boosts gut and brain health and protects against diabetes, heart disease, and cancer.

- Beans are particularly beneficial to gut health. They fuel the growth of beneficial bacteria in the upper digestive tract, and the high amount of resistant starch and fiber they contain means that not all calories from beans are absorbed by the body and instead help to pull fats from the bottom of the digestive tract.

- Eating beans at one meal also helps to improve your insulin response to high-glycemic foods in subsequent meals, giving you better glycemic control at meals for the rest of the day. Some studies have found this amazing effect (known as the "second-meal effect") persisting to the following day.

- Studies have shown that people who eat beans regularly enjoy lower blood pressure, cholesterol, and inflammation, as well as higher fiber and mineral intake, and are less likely to be overweight than those who don't frequently eat beans.

CLASSIC HUMMUS

Undoubtedly the most popular recipe on my blog, this no-oil hummus gets its creaminess from aquafaba, the liquid from a can of chickpeas. Aquafaba also helps add smoothness and viscosity without the calories of olive oil. This hummus is creamy, tangy, and always found in my fridge!

MAKES ABOUT 3 CUPS (TWELVE ¼-CUP OR NINE ⅓-CUP SERVINGS)

2⅔ cups canned chickpeas (see Note), drained, ¾ cup of their liquid (aquafaba) reserved
¼ cup tahini
¼ cup lemon juice
1½ tablespoons white miso paste
½ teaspoon garlic powder
1 teaspoon ground cumin

Combine all the ingredients in a high-speed blender and blend on high until smooth and creamy, 60 to 90 seconds. Serve immediately or transfer to a storage container.

Storage: Store in the fridge in a glass food storage container or glass jar with a tight-fitting lid for at least 10 days.

Enjoy!

My all-time favorite way to enjoy this hummus is as a healthful and flavorful salad dressing (try it on the Simple Rainbow Hummus Salad on page 178). You can also make a delicious, super-quick creamed kale by adding this hummus to a batch of Simple Sautéed Greens (page 246). Or use it as a better-for-you baked potato topping, for crudités, or as a sauce for whole-grain and vegetable bowls.

Notes: Some stores carry cooked beans packaged in shelf-stable cartons (I buy cartons of Whole Foods 365 brand beans); these can be used in place of canned beans. You can also cook dried beans from scratch and use those instead (just be sure to save enough of the cooking liquid to substitute for the aquafaba); either option will work for this recipe.
- The white miso paste really makes this hummus special, adding a unique salty, umami flavor and probiotic health benefits. If you can't find white miso paste, you can add salt to taste; just note that the flavor will be quite different.

BEET HUMMUS

Pink and fuchsia foods are my personal favorites, and that's why you'll always see bright pops of these colors in my fridge. I didn't always love beets (I used to think they tasted like dirt), but after making them a regular part of my health transformation, I've grown to love them. Now I add fresh or roasted beets to all the things, and this slightly sweet, earthy, no-oil hummus really lets that beet flavor shine!

MAKES ABOUT 2 CUPS (EIGHT ¼-CUP SERVINGS)

1⅓ cups canned chickpeas, drained, ¼ cup of their liquid (aquafaba) reserved (see Note, page 197)
¾ cup chopped cooked red beets (such as Classic Roasted Beets, page 252)
¼ cup tahini
2 tablespoons lemon juice
1 tablespoon balsamic vinegar
⅛ teaspoon garlic powder

Combine all the ingredients in a high-speed blender and blend on high until smooth and creamy, 60 to 90 seconds. Serve immediately or transfer to storage containers.

Storage: Store in the fridge in a glass food storage container or glass jar with a tight-fitting lid for up to 10 days.

Note: If you're new to plant-based eating, I recommend starting out with the Classic Hummus recipe first.

ITALIAN HERB CANNELLINI BEAN HUMMUS

I love the rich flavor combination of cannellini beans and protein-rich raw pine nuts with the freshness of the herbs in this Italian-inspired recipe. If you follow a plant-based diet, you can even think of it as an ultra-healthy herbed "faux-cotta cheese."

MAKES 2½ CUPS (TEN ¼-CUP SERVINGS)

2½ cups canned cannellini beans, drained, ¼ cup of their liquid (aquafaba) reserved (see Note, page 197)
¼ cup raw pine nuts
2 tablespoons nutritional yeast
1 tablespoon lemon juice
¼ to ½ teaspoon salt
⅓ cup Classic Vegan Parmesan (page 190)
½ cup chopped fresh basil
2 tablespoons chopped fresh parsley
1 teaspoon dried oregano
Ground black pepper

Combine the beans, aquafaba, pine nuts, nutritional yeast, lemon juice, and salt in a high-speed blender and blend on high until smooth and creamy, 60 to 90 seconds.

Scrape the hummus into a bowl. Fold in the vegan parmesan, basil, parsley, and oregano and season with pepper to taste. Serve immediately or transfer to storage containers.

Storage: Store in the fridge in a glass food storage container or glass jar with a tight-fitting lid for up to 10 days.

Enjoy!

I love dolloping this hummus on top of Garden Veggie Minestrone Soup (page 228), Quick and Crispy Spinach and Artichoke Flatbreads (page 320), and Spaghetti and Meatball Prep Bowls (page 292), especially when I want something more substantial than just a sprinkling of Classic Vegan Parmesan (page 190).

Note: I don't recommend trying this hummus recipe if you're brand new to vegan, whole-food eating. If you wanted to make this a bit more approachable, you could stir in ½ to 1 tablespoon olive oil after blending.

PUMPKIN HUMMUS

I remember stopping dead in my tracks at the grocery store when I first saw sweet hummuses. With flavors like pumpkin, chocolate, and even cookie dough, I was so excited to try them, until I checked the label and saw all the added sugar and oil. I went straight home and started developing this recipe, and it was love at first bite! To me, this pumpkin hummus tastes about as close as you can get to whole-food plant-based pumpkin pie filling (which is always my favorite part of the pie anyway).

MAKES 2½ CUPS (TEN ¼-CUP SERVINGS)

1⅓ cups no-added-salt chickpeas, drained and rinsed

1 cup canned pure pumpkin puree

¼ cup raw cashews

6 Medjool dates, pitted, or 2 tablespoons maple syrup

¼ cup almond milk or your favorite plant milk, plus more if needed

¼ teaspoon vanilla powder or vanilla extract, or seeds from ½ vanilla bean

½ teaspoon ground cinnamon

⅛ teaspoon ground nutmeg

⅛ teaspoon ground ginger

Combine all the ingredients in a high-speed blender and blend on high until smooth and creamy, 60 to 90 seconds. You may need to use your tamper or stop and scrape down the sides if your blender jar is wider than 4 inches. Add up to 1 tablespoon additional almond milk as needed to reach the desired creaminess. Serve immediately or transfer to storage containers.

Storage: Store in the fridge in a glass food storage container or glass jar with a tight-fitting lid for up to 10 days.

Enjoy!

My son, hubby, and I love using this as a dip for fresh fall apples. I also use it in Easy Autumn Parfaits (page 327). And I like to make an autumn pita pizza by toasting the pita in the oven, then using this hummus as a base and topping it with sliced apples, pomegranates, and dried cranberries.

Note: You won't use the whole can of pumpkin for this recipe, but you can use the leftover portion for Pumpkin Spice Cashew Creamer (page 307).

CHOCOLATE HUMMUS

You may be surprised to see black beans in a dessert, but they serve as the perfect low-fat base to create this decadent, chocolate-pudding-like hummus that even my twelve-year-old chocoholic can't get enough of!

MAKES ABOUT 2 CUPS (EIGHT ¼-CUP SERVINGS)

1¼ cups no-added-salt black beans, drained and rinsed
8 Medjool dates, pitted and coarsely chopped
½ cup plus 2 tablespoons vanilla almond milk or your favorite plant milk
¼ cup unsweetened cocoa powder
2 tablespoons ground flaxseed
½ teaspoon vanilla powder or vanilla extract, or seeds from 1 vanilla bean
¼ teaspoon ground cinnamon

Combine all the ingredients in a high-speed blender and blend on high until smooth and creamy, 60 to 90 seconds. The hummus will have a shiny, fluffy, pudding-like consistency. Serve immediately or transfer to storage containers.

Storage: Store in the fridge in a glass food storage container or glass jar with a tight-fitting lid for up to 10 days.

Enjoy!

I love eating this hummus with fresh bananas, strawberries, raspberries, and pomegranates. I'll add it to warm oatmeal bowls (this hummus tastes amazing warmed, too) for a special treat. It's also used as a base for Easy Chocolate Parfaits (page 327).

Note: If you're using canned black beans, you'll have some left over—use them in a Mexican Quinoa Casserole (page 268) or store them in the fridge as part of your in-fridge salad bar toppings stash (see page 177).

BLENDED OR CHOPPED CONDIMENTS

Tasty, healthy sauces and other condiments are such an easy way to enhance cooked veggies, prep bowls, soups, and salads. Because these recipes are dairy-free, they enjoy superior shelf life in your fridge, so you can easily mix and match them with your other preps for the week.

NACHO CHEESE SAUCE

This is my liquid gold! I can't tell you how many bowls of steamed broccoli, sautéed spinach, bean pastas, and baked potatoes I've enjoyed topped with this sauce. This creamy, velvety, savory cheese sauce is consistently one of the most well-loved and reviewed recipes on my site—making believers out of omnivores and vegans alike!

MAKES 2¾ CUPS (ELEVEN ¼-CUP SERVINGS)

1½ cups raw cashews, soaked overnight, if desired (see Note)
1 (12-ounce) jar roasted red peppers (not packed in oil), drained
¾ cup water
½ cup nutritional yeast
3 tablespoons lemon juice
2 teaspoons onion powder
¼ teaspoon garlic powder
¼ to ½ teaspoon salt

Combine all the ingredients in a high-speed blender (see Notes). Blend on high for 1½ to 2 minutes, until the sauce is very smooth and creamy and warmed from the high-speed blending. It's okay if you see steam building up inside the blender jar.

If you're making nachos, I like to pour the warmed sauce over the chips right out of the blender. Or let cool completely before transferring to storage containers.

Storage: Store in the fridge in a glass food container or jar on an upper shelf for 9 to 12 days or freeze for up to 2 months. Bring it to room temperature, then warm it up in a small pot over medium-low heat, using a whisk to reincorporate. If the sauce looks particularly watery, cook until it condenses.

Enjoy!

Create the ultimate loaded vegan nachos by using this sauce on Oil-Free Tortilla Chips (page 232) or your favorite chips. I love tossing this with al dente pasta shells or rotini. It's also amazing on a bowl of lightly steamed purple fingerling potatoes or red potatoes and lightly steamed broccoli, topped with sliced green onions. This cheese sauce is a main ingredient in the Mexican Quinoa Casserole (page 268).

Notes:

- It's up to you if you want to soak the cashews overnight before blending. It makes a slightly creamier sauce, but I usually make this sauce without soaking. If your blender is a less powerful model, soaking will make it easier to break down the cashews.
- The sauce will thicken in the fridge, but generally thins out when reheated in the microwave or on the stovetop. If it is still too thick after reheating, whisk in a bit of water.
- For a spicier queso-like flavor, replace the lemon juice with lime juice and add 1 teaspoon ground chipotle pepper or your favorite chili powder.

CLASSIC VEGAN PARMESAN

This parmesan is known in the vegan world as "fairy dust," because you just want to go around sprinkling it on all the things! Incredibly easy to make, this cheese-like condiment is a staple in my fridge because it has such an incredible shelf life and adds so much savory, cheesy flavor and umami to our soups, pastas, flatbread pizzas, and salads.

MAKES ABOUT 2 CUPS (SIXTEEN 2-TABLESPOON SERVINGS)

1¼ cups raw cashews
½ cup nutritional yeast
½ teaspoon garlic powder
½ teaspoon salt, plus more if needed

Combine all the ingredients in a high-speed blender. Blend on high for 10 seconds, then stop and scrape down the sides. Blend for 5 to 7 seconds more, then check the consistency—the texture should be crumbly; a few larger pieces of cashew here and there are okay and will add a bit of texture. Do not overblend.

Storage: Store in the fridge in a 1-pint glass jar with a tight-fitting lid for up to 3 months.

Enjoy!

You'll find this vegan parmesan used in Italian Herb Cannellini Bean Hummus (page 185), Kale Caesar Salad Jars (page 297), Spinach and Artichoke Dip (page 242), and Quick and Crispy Spinach and Artichoke Flatbreads (page 320).

SWEET-AND-SOUR SAUCE

Who's ready for an amazingly flavorful sweet-and-sour sauce without loads of sugar and oil? This recipe uses the unique thickening properties of dates, as well as their natural sweetness, to make an authentic-tasting sweet-and-sour sauce in your blender.

MAKES ABOUT 1½ CUPS (SIX ¼-CUP SERVINGS)

1 to 2 tablespoons canned crushed pineapple (see Notes), plus ½ cup juice from the can
4 Medjool dates, pitted and coarsely chopped
¼ cup tomato paste
3 tablespoons rice vinegar
2 garlic cloves, minced or pressed
1 to 2 teaspoons minced fresh ginger, to taste (see Notes)
1 tablespoon tamari
¼ cup roasted red pepper (about 1 pepper), drained and rinsed
¼ teaspoon red pepper flakes

Combine the pineapple juice, dates, tomato paste, vinegar, garlic, ginger, and tamari in a high-speed blender (see Notes). Blend on high for 30 to 40 seconds, until smooth. Add the roasted pepper and blend for 5 seconds more, or until the pepper is broken down into little bits but still visible.

Add the crushed pineapple and red pepper flakes to the blender and blend to combine, or pour the sauce into a bowl and stir in the pineapple and red pepper flakes.

Storage: Store in the fridge in a glass food storage container or glass jar with a tight-fitting lid for 9 to 12 days.

Enjoy!

I love tossing this sauce with pasta and lightly steamed broccoli, and it's a main component in the Sweet-and-Sour Meatball Prep Bowls (page 290), one of my favorite meals in this book! You could also use it as a dipping sauce for Rainbow Collard Wraps (page 322). This sauce pairs well with plant-based proteins and animal proteins alike.

Notes:
- The leftover canned pineapple can be used to make Decadent Tropical Coconut Chia Pudding (page 219).
- If you find fresh ginger too strong a flavor, start with 1 teaspoon and add more if you like.
- You can use a regular blender for this recipe if your dates are soft and moist. If they are on the drier/harder side, soak them in hot water for 10 minutes and then drain before blending.

CLEANEST MAYO

There are store-bought vegan mayonnaise brands on the market, but they all list oil within the first three ingredients. This whole-food alternative gets its creaminess from cashews instead.

MAKES ABOUT 2 CUPS (EIGHT ¼-CUP SERVINGS)

1½ cups raw cashews, soaked overnight (see Note)
3 tablespoons lemon juice
1 tablespoon apple cider vinegar
¾ to 1 teaspoon salt
¾ cup water

Drain and rinse the cashews. Combine the cashews, lemon juice, vinegar, salt, and water in a high-speed blender and blend on high for about 60 seconds, until smooth and creamy.

The mayo will have better flavor and texture after 1 day in the fridge.

Storage: Store in the fridge in a 1-pint glass jar with a tight-fitting lid for 10 to 12 days, or up to 14 days if stored on a top shelf toward the back, near an airflow source, and condensed into smaller jars as it is used.

Enjoy!

This is a perfect sandwich spread and is used as a base for Vegan Ranch Dressing (page 195), Classic Chickpea Salad (page 214), Vegan Egg Salad (page 216), and Spinach and Artichoke Dip (page 242).

Notes:

- Soaking raw cashews gives this mayo the creamiest texture and the best flavor. I like to soak them in a widemouthed quart-size glass jar overnight, then drain them and rinse with cool running water.
- For a spicy chipotle-flavored mayo, replace the lemon juice with lime juice, omit the vinegar, and add 1 teaspoon ground chipotle pepper or canned chipotle in adobo sauce.

FRESH PICO DE GALLO

Nothing is more refreshingly delicious than peak-season pico de gallo. While I'll still buy pre-made pico de gallo in the winter and spring months, taking a bit of extra time to make it at home with ripe in-season tomatoes gives you complete control over sodium levels and spiciness. I like to make this without any added salt because heirloom tomatoes have so much natural depth of flavor.

MAKES ABOUT 3 CUPS (TWELVE ¼-CUP SERVINGS)

1¾ cups diced fresh tomatoes (preferably heirloom)
¾ cup diced red onion (about ½ large)
¼ cup finely diced jalapeño (about 1 large, most seeds removed)
¼ cup chopped fresh cilantro
3 tablespoons lime juice
1 tablespoon minced or pressed garlic (about 3 large cloves)
Salt and ground black pepper

In a medium bowl, stir together the tomatoes, onion, jalapeño, cilantro, lime juice, and garlic. Season with salt and pepper and allow to sit for at least 10 minutes before serving.

Storage: Store in the fridge in a glass food storage container or glass jars with a tight-fitting lid for up to 10 days.

Enjoy!

This makes an amazing salad dressing for black beans, brown rice, corn, and fresh avocado over a bed of romaine. I also love using it as a topping for baked potatoes, on nachos, or on pasta tossed with Nacho Cheese Sauce (page 188). It's also used as a component in Mexican Quinoa Casserole (page 268), Taco Salad Jars (page 303), and Easy Taco Sliders (page 324).

QUICK PANTRY SALSA

This recipe started off as a trick I learned from my sister-in-law, Julie, for when you're clean out of fresh salsa ingredients and you don't want to (or can't) head out to the store. It was a boon to my family in the early days of the COVID-19 pandemic, when it was hard to get groceries delivered and fresh produce was particularly difficult to find. My hubby and I happily lived off this pantry salsa for several weeks—it tastes just as good as the fresh stuff!

MAKES JUST OVER 3 CUPS (TWELVE ¼-CUP SERVINGS)

2 (14.5-ounce) cans fire-roasted diced tomatoes (with or without green chiles)
1 canned chipotle pepper in adobo sauce, plus 1 tablespoon sauce from the can (or to taste)
½ teaspoon salt
1 tablespoon dried cilantro, or ½ cup chopped fresh cilantro (optional)
1 tablespoon onion granules or freeze-dried red onion (optional)
1 to 2 tablespoons lime juice (optional)

Combine the tomatoes, chipotle pepper, adobo sauce, and salt in a blender and blend on medium speed for about 10 seconds, until the chipotle is well incorporated but the salsa still has a slightly chunky texture. Add the cilantro, onion, and/or lime juice, if desired (or if you have them on hand), and pulse 3 or 4 times, until just incorporated and chopped a little. Taste and adjust the seasonings to your liking.

Storage: Store in the fridge in a glass food storage container or glass jars with a tight-fitting lid for 12 to 14 days.

Enjoy!

Use this salsa just as you would any other salsa or hot sauce. I love eating this over quinoa, brown rice, or cauliflower rice with Tofu Taco Meat (page 273), corn, black beans, finely shredded lettuce, and avocado, with a drizzle of Nacho Cheese Sauce (page 188).

Note: If you want more of a hot sauce consistency, blend everything on high speed until very smooth.

VEGAN RANCH DRESSING

This iteration of the classic creamy salad dressing boasts plenty of tangy, herby flavor—you'll be amazed at just how much this healthier version tastes like the "real thing."

MAKES 1¾ CUPS (SEVEN ¼-CUP SERVINGS)

1½ cups vegan mayo, homemade (page 192) or store-bought (see Note)
¼ cup unsweetened almond milk, or more as needed (see Note)
1½ teaspoons nutritional yeast
1 teaspoon apple cider vinegar
3 garlic cloves, pressed or minced
1½ teaspoons dried parsley
1 teaspoon dried dill
1 teaspoon onion powder
¼ teaspoon paprika
Salt and ground black pepper

In a medium bowl, whisk together the mayo, almond milk, nutritional yeast, vinegar, garlic, parsley, dill, onion powder, and paprika. Season with salt and pepper. If the dressing is too thick, adjust the consistency to your preference by whisking in more almond milk.

Transfer to a storage container or jar and refrigerate for at least a few hours or preferably overnight before using to let the flavors meld.

Storage: Store in the fridge in a glass food storage container or glass jars with a tight-fitting lid(s) for 7 to 9 days.

Enjoy!

My hubby and I enjoy this drizzled over rainbow salads (see page 295), as a sauce for summer potato salads, or mixed with pasta elbows and fresh-cut bell peppers, carrots, and celery for a BBQ-friendly side dish.

Note: You can substitute egg-based mayo for vegan mayo and/or dairy milk for the almond milk, but note that the shelf life will decrease to 3 to 5 days.

CASHEW CAESAR DRESSING

While away on a work trip not long after going vegan, I went to my very first vegan restaurant. It was an eye-opening experience, especially when they brought out a giant Caesar salad that tasted exactly like the real thing! With each creamy, savory bite, I became more and more convinced that so many more people would choose to go vegan if they could enjoy food this delicious. This dressing recipe was inspired by that pivotal experience. Note that the kelp granules are optional, but they help mimic the briny flavor of the anchovies in traditional Caesar dressing.

MAKES ABOUT 2 CUPS (EIGHT ¼-CUP SERVINGS)

1¼ cups raw cashews
¾ cup water
2 teaspoons Dijon mustard
2 tablespoons lemon juice
2 tablespoons tahini
1 tablespoon apple cider vinegar
1 tablespoon capers (some brine is okay)
2 garlic cloves, peeled
2 teaspoons white miso paste
½ teaspoon kelp granules (optional)
Salt and ground black pepper
1 to 2 tablespoons unsweetened almond milk (optional)

Combine the cashews, water, mustard, lemon juice, tahini, vinegar, capers, garlic, miso, and kelp granules (if using) in a high-speed blender. Season with salt and pepper and blend on high for 1½ minutes, or until smooth and creamy. This dressing is very thick and gets thicker after it's stored in the fridge, so you can thin it by blending in plain, unsweetened almond milk until it reaches your desired texture.

Storage: Store in the fridge in a 1-pint glass jar or glass food storage container with a tight-fitting lid for 10 to 12 days.

Enjoy!

I love eating this Caesar dressing with all kinds of cooked and fresh veggies—it works wonderfully as a dip, especially when you keep the texture thicker. You'll use this dressing in the Kale Caesar Salad Jars (page 297). I also love tossing it with roasted or braised baby Broccolini for a beautifully refined side dish that can please a crowd of different eaters!

ZESTY OIL-FREE AQUAFABA ITALIAN DRESSING

When I was a little girl, I remember my mom making homemade Italian dressing in a tall glass cruet. She'd add the oil and vinegar and the spice packet, close the white plastic lid, and shake, shake, shake. I used to love watching all the specks swirl and settle to the bottom. This is my healthy, plant-based Italian dressing in that spirit. The secret-weapon ingredient is aquafaba, the liquid from canned chickpeas, which gives the dressing richness and body thanks to its natural proteins and starches.

MAKES ABOUT 1¾ CUPS (SEVEN ¼-CUP SERVINGS)

1¼ cups aquafaba (see Notes)

3 tablespoons distilled white vinegar

1 tablespoon chia seeds, preferably white chia

1 tablespoon nutritional yeast

1 teaspoon Dijon mustard

¼ teaspoon salt

½ teaspoon minced or pressed garlic

1 to 1½ teaspoons Italian seasoning

¼ to ½ teaspoon red pepper flakes

Combine the aquafaba, vinegar, chia, nutritional yeast, mustard, and salt in a high-speed blender (see Notes). Blend for 20 seconds, or until smooth.

Pour into a glass jar or glass food storage container and stir in the garlic, Italian seasoning, and red pepper flakes to combine (do not blend). Cover and refrigerate overnight before eating. The dressing will be quite frothy right out of the blender, but it will settle and thicken as it chills.

Storage: Store in the fridge in a glass food storage container or glass jar with a tight-fitting lid for 7 to 9 days.

Notes:

- The amount of aquafaba in a can of chickpeas varies from just less than 1 cup to 1⅓ cups, depending on the brand. You may need one or two 15.5-ounce cans to get enough for this recipe. You can use the chickpeas in Pumpkin Hummus (page 186), Classic Chickpea Salad (page 214) or Classic Roasted Chickpeas (page 279).
- If you have a high-speed blender with a larger base, this recipe may not blend well for you. If that's the case, you can whisk together all the ingredients in a bowl. Just note that the look of the dressing will be different and the consistency will be looser. You can add another 1½ teaspoons chia seeds to help thicken it, if desired.

FRIDGE PICKLES

I was introduced to the wonderful world of quick pickling when I first joined the vegan community on Instagram. I was entranced by the beautiful, vibrant color of pickled red onion and red cabbage and had already learned that vinegar was a wonderful salt substitute when eating a low-sodium diet.

I started experimenting on my own, and now I eat fridge-pickled veggies every day. They instantly lift the flavor of the foods you add them to, have a terrific crunchy texture, and require no cooking at all! Quick pickling is such a simple technique to make your everyday meals feel more special and look beautiful.

FRIDGE PICKLE TECHNIQUE

Step 1: Select your veggies—the more darkly pigmented, the better (this means they're more nutritious and will also produce the best color). Red cabbage, red onion, radishes, and shredded beets create the most beautiful and vivid orange, red, pink, and purple colors. But carrots, cucumbers, and even beet stems all work well with this technique.

Step 2: Cut your veggies. This is all up to your preference. You can choose a very thin slice or a dice—either works.

Step 3: Select your jar(s). Keep in mind that it will need to be large enough to hold both the veggies and the pickling brine.

Step 4: Make your brine, choosing one of the recipes that follow.

Step 5: Pack your jar(s). Start by placing the prepped veggies in the jar. Add a halved garlic clove, if desired, or even fresh herbs or your favorite spices, then pour in the brine; as a general rule, you want the brine to fill the jar to no more than 1 inch from the top of the jar. Seal the jar with a lid and refrigerate.

Step 6: The waiting game. I wouldn't recommend eating the pickles within the first 24 hours, because the vinegar flavor is most potent at this stage. You want to give your pickles enough time to get flavorful and properly colored—for red cabbage and shredded beets, that's about 48 hours, and for red onions and radishes, it's about 3 days. If the brine doesn't completely cover the veggies, it's a good idea to give the container an occasional quick shake in the first few days to help distribute the pickling liquid.

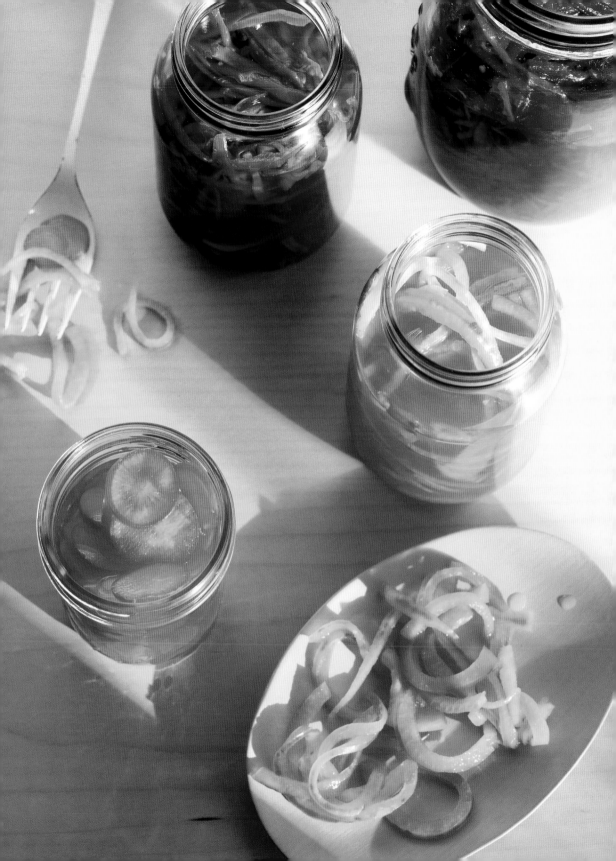

Storage: Note that these are called fridge pickles because they are made and stored in the fridge; they are not canned for long-term storage or storage at room temperature. But fridge pickles do have a wonderfully long shelf life! Stored in a glass jar (my favorite storage method) or glass food storage container with a tight-fitting lid, most will keep for a minimum of 3 to 4 weeks (I frequently have batches that stay fresh and delicious for almost 3 months). Fridge pickles made with cucumbers will keep for 7 to 9 days.

Notes:
- Sometimes I'll add a small chunk of raw or roasted beets to my pickled red onions and radishes to amplify their pink color!
- I love drizzling the leftover pickling liquid over my oil-free hummuses (pages 183–187).

Enjoy!

My hubby and I eat fridge pickles at almost every savory meal! They're perfect in salads, bowls, tacos, and tofu scrambles and on top of soups. You'll see them used in many of the recipes in this book.

EASIEST BRINE

This is the brine I used to make my fridge pickles when I first got started, and it's still my favorite! I happen to love a strong vinegar flavor and prefer not to add salt to foods when I can help it. If you're new to fridge pickles, I would recommend starting off with one of the other brines first—this one is easiest, but it also has the strongest vinegar flavor. If desired, you can replace half the vinegar with water.

Cut vegetables (best for this brine: red onion, red cabbage, or radishes)
Garlic, halved (optional)
Distilled white vinegar
Water (optional)

Add your cut vegetables and optional garlic to your container and cover with vinegar (or half water and half vinegar).

SAVORY BRINE

This brine strikes a lovely balance between salt and vinegar, and the added water helps to keep the vinegar flavor tamed. If you are new to fridge pickles, I highly recommend starting with this brine!

MAKES ¾ CUP

½ cup distilled white vinegar
¼ cup water
¼ teaspoon salt
Sprinkle of garlic powder, or ½ garlic clove (optional)
About 1 cup prepped veggies

In a small bowl, whisk together the vinegar, water, salt, and garlic powder (if using). Place the veggies in a 1-pint glass jar and add the garlic clove (if using). Pour the brine over the veggies and mix to incorporate if the brine doesn't reach the top of the jar.

SWEET BRINE

Maple syrup is the perfect complement to apple cider vinegar and helps bring a mellow, balanced flavor to fridge pickles, without the need for added salt.

MAKES ¾ CUP

½ cup apple cider vinegar
1½ tablespoons maple syrup
¼ cup water
Sprinkle of garlic powder, or ½ garlic clove (optional)
About 1 cup prepped veggies

In a small bowl, whisk together the vinegar, maple syrup, water, and garlic powder (if using). Place the veggies in a 1-pint glass jar and add the garlic clove (if using). Pour the brine over the veggies and mix to incorporate if the brine doesn't reach the top of the jar.

APPLE CIDER VINEGAR AND MINT SHREDDED BEETS

I love the flavor combination of mint and beets; I find that the fresh mint complements the beets' natural earthiness. I like to make this recipe when I'm also making Quinoa Tabouleh (page 261), another recipe that calls for fresh mint. The brine from these pickles is my favorite to drizzle over Simple Rainbow Hummus Salad (page 178) when I need a change from my normal balsamic vinegar.

MAKES 2 CUPS

2 medium beets, trimmed and peeled with a vegetable peeler (see Note)
½ cup apple cider vinegar
¼ cup water
½ teaspoon salt
1 teaspoon maple syrup
1 to 2 tablespoons finely chopped fresh mint
Sprinkle of garlic powder, or ½ garlic clove (optional)

Shred the beets. (I like to use my food processor attachment for this; quarter each beet first so they'll fit through the feeder attachment.) Set aside.

In a large bowl, whisk together the vinegar, water, salt, maple syrup, mint, and garlic powder (if using). Add the shredded beets to the bowl and stir to combine with the brine.

Spoon into a 1-pint glass jar and add the garlic clove (if using). These are best enjoyed after at least 24 hours in the fridge.

Storage: Store in the fridge in a glass jar or glass food storage container with a tight-fitting lid for 3 to 4 weeks (or longer).

Note: One of the recipe testers for this book, Gail, used cooked beets and loved the results—so you can opt for cooked if that's what you have on hand.

SMOOTHIE FREEZER PACKS

Making weekly smoothie packs is a prepping mainstay for a reason—it works! Taking the time to portion out your ingredients means you can just grab a smoothie pack, add liquid, blend, and go.

For the three recipes I've included here, each smoothie pack makes one serving; you can scale them up however you like. I use the smoothie attachment for my Vitamix Ascent series blender, but if you have a high-speed blender with a wider-based jar, blending an individual portion might not work. If that's the case, I recommend doubling the recipes and, after blending, sharing the smoothie with someone or storing the second serving in the fridge for later (see Storage, page 204).

If your blender is having trouble breaking down the frozen smoothie packs, you can follow a tip from Kim, one of my recipe testers, who has a basic Vitamix model. She found that letting the smoothie pack thaw a bit before blending helped make a smooth consistency. You can also add more liquid for better blending.

Step 1: Put your fresh smoothie ingredients in a plastic or silicone storage bag. You can include fresh fruit, leafy greens like kale or spinach, and even nuts, seeds, and pitted dates (just make sure to chop them before freezing to help your blender later). Label the bag (it's also a nice idea to write the type and amount of liquid you'll need for the smoothie right on the bag to help you remember).

Step 2: Freeze the bag at least overnight before using the contents to make a smoothie.

Step 3: When you're ready to blend, transfer the contents of the smoothie pack to a high-speed blender and add the recommended liquid. Blend on high speed until smooth.

Storage: Smoothie packs will keep in the freezer for up to 2 months, but freezer burn can become an issue. It's a good idea to place individual bags into a larger airtight plastic container to minimize freezer burn. I like to store leftover blended smoothies in a glass jar with a tight-fitting lid on an upper shelf at the far back of my fridge, as close as I can get to the airflow source. Stored this way, they will keep for up to 4 days. Note that the texture will become more like a juice after 12 hours.

Enjoy!

Make smoothies for your breakfast, as an afternoon pick-me-up (my kids love these), or as a healthy dessert!

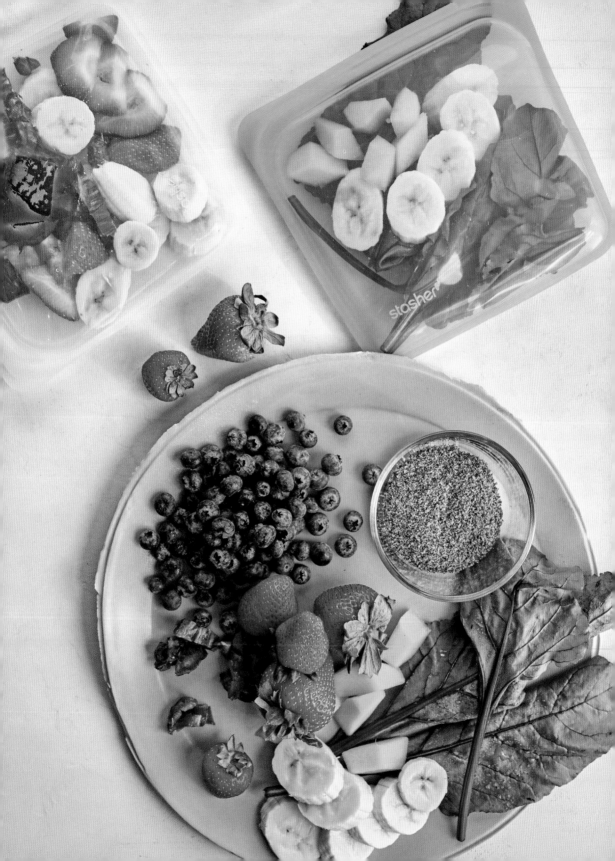

CLASSIC GREEN SMOOTHIE

When you have a green smoothie for breakfast, you're breaking your body's night-time fast with the highest-nutrient veggies in the world—providing your body with amazing energy right from the day's start. The key is to use just enough fruit to combat the bitterness from the greens. As you get more accustomed to the taste, challenge yourself to go darker and darker green by adding more leafy greens!

MAKES 1 SMOOTHIE (ABOUT 1⅔ CUPS)

Place in plastic or silicone baggie

½ banana, sliced

½ cup plus 2 tablespoons frozen or fresh sweet fruit (like pineapple or mango or a combo)

1 packed cup fresh or frozen greens (such as kale, spinach, chard, and/or beet greens)

1½ teaspoons ground flaxseed

1 Medjool date, pitted and chopped (optional)

Add when blending

¾ cup unsweetened coconut water (see Note)

Combine the banana, sweet fruit, greens, flaxseed, and date (if using) in a plastic or silicone storage bag. Seal and store in the freezer overnight or until ready to use, up to 2 months.

To make your smoothie, grab the smoothie pack from the freezer, empty the contents into a high-speed blender, add the coconut water, and blend on high until smooth and creamy, 60 to 90 seconds.

Note: You can adjust the sweetness of the recipe to your desired level; including the date and using sweetened coconut water will result in a sweeter smoothie.

BLUEBERRY SMOOTHIE

Blueberries are one of the healthiest fruits you can eat. They're low in calories (with a significantly lower sugar content than other fruits) and incredibly rich in antioxidants and phytonutrients. This smoothie is a real winner in my household because of its gorgeous light purple color and simple ingredients. My kids absolutely love this smoothie as an afternoon snack, and I enjoy it for dessert when I'm craving something sweet but don't want anything too rich.

MAKES 1 SMOOTHIE (1⅔ CUPS)

Place in plastic or silicone baggie

½ banana, sliced
¾ cup frozen or fresh blueberries
1 tablespoon flaxseed
1 Medjool date, pitted and chopped (optional; see Note)

Add when blending

1 cup vanilla almond milk

Combine the banana, blueberries, flaxseed, and date (if using) in a plastic or silicone storage bag. Seal and store in the freezer overnight or until ready to use, up to 2 months.

To make your smoothie, grab the smoothie pack from the freezer, empty the contents into a high-speed blender, add the almond milk, and blend on high until smooth, 60 to 90 seconds.

Notes:

- This is not a thick smoothie; it's almost like an infused almond milk to me, but it's a consistency my family really enjoys.
- Instead of the date, you could use 1 tablespoon maple syrup; add it with the almond milk before blending.
- When blueberries are out of season, they can be quite tart; adding a date (or maple syrup—see above) and/or using sweetened almond milk can help balance that tartness. If your berries are sweeter, you may want to omit the sweeteners.

BEET-BERRY SMOOTHIE

I never pass up an opportunity to enjoy naturally pink foods—they just make me smile! This smoothie is extra amazing because not only is it a beautifully bright fuchsia color, it's also loaded with betalains, phytonutrients that reduce inflammation and protect against oxidative damage to cells. If you're a little intimidated by the flavor of beets, this recipe is a great way to enjoy them, since they're paired with sweet fruits.

MAKES 1 SMOOTHIE (JUST OVER 1½ CUPS)

Place in plastic or silicone baggie

½ very spotty banana, sliced

½ cup plus 2 tablespoons chopped cooked red beets (such as Classic Roasted Beets, page 252)

4 large fresh or frozen strawberries

2 Medjool dates, pitted and chopped

Add when blending

1 cup vanilla almond milk (see Notes)

Combine the banana, beets, strawberries, and dates in a plastic or silicone storage bag. Seal and store in the freezer overnight or until ready to use, up to 2 months.

To make your smoothie, grab the smoothie pack from the freezer, empty the contents into a high-speed blender, add the almond milk, and blend on high until smooth and creamy, 60 to 90 seconds.

Notes:

- If you're new to plant-based eating, this flavor combination may be something you will want to work up to. I suggest starting with one of the other smoothie pack recipes first.
- I prefer unsweetened almond milk, but use sweetened if you like.

OVERNIGHT OATS

These are an absolute meal-prepping must because they're so darn easy to make. Over the past year, I've recruited my kids into prepping these for the whole family for the week in the warmer months. It's a fun activity we usually do after dinner on Sundays—my daughter is notorious for sneaking bites and getting almost halfway into her Monday jar before it ever hits the fridge!

These are so simple, in fact, that I recommend new preppers start by just prepping this one item for breakfast for the week. I've included two classic flavors and one more advanced recipe for when you're ready for something a bit more involved. You can scale up the recipes as needed depending on how many people you're feeding and how many days you want to prep for at once.

Storage: These oatmeal dishes should be stored in the fridge in glass food storage containers or glass jars with tight-fitting lids and will keep for 5 to 7 days. If you're going to batch prep these for the week, I recommend storing some of them on the top shelf toward the back of your fridge, as this typically extends shelf life the most.

VANILLA OVERNIGHT OATS

This is the basic recipe I think every meal prepper should have in their repertoire. It's sweetened with just banana (my kids enjoy it this way), but you could certainly add maple syrup to taste if you wish!

MAKES ABOUT 2 CUPS (2 SERVINGS), DEPENDING ON THE SIZE OF THE BANANA

1 ripe, spotty banana (the more speckled the skin, the sweeter the banana)
¼ teaspoon vanilla powder or vanilla extract, or seeds from 1 vanilla bean (optional)
¼ teaspoon ground cinnamon (optional)
1 cup rolled oats
2 tablespoons chia seeds
1 cup unsweetened almond milk

In a medium bowl, mash the banana with a fork or potato masher. Add the vanilla and/or cinnamon (if using) and combine well. Add the oats, chia seeds, and almond milk and mix well.

Divide the mixture between glass food storage containers or glass jars and seal with their lids. Refrigerate for at least 6 hours or preferably overnight before eating.

Storage: Store in the fridge in glass food storage containers or glass jars with tight-fitting lids for 5 to 7 days.

Enjoy!

My whole family enjoys these as is, but sometimes we like to jazz things up with different fresh toppings. Sliced bananas, fresh berries, fridge jams (pages 253–258), and nut butters go really well with this recipe.

PUMPKIN OVERNIGHT OATS

These seasonal oats feature canned pumpkin puree in lieu of mashed banana. Because pumpkin isn't naturally very sweet, a bit of maple syrup adds sweetness and a lovely autumn flavor to these oats.

MAKES ABOUT 2 CUPS (TWO 1-CUP SERVINGS)

1 cup rolled oats

1 cup unsweetened almond milk or your favorite plant milk

½ cup canned pure pumpkin puree

2 tablespoons maple syrup

2 tablespoons chia seeds

½ to 1 teaspoon ground cinnamon

1/16 teaspoon ground nutmeg (optional)

Combine all the ingredients in a medium bowl. Divide the mixture between glass food storage containers or glass jars and seal with their lids. Refrigerate for at least 6 hours or preferably overnight before eating.

Storage: Store in the fridge in glass food storage containers or glass jars with tight-fitting lids for 5 to 7 days.

Enjoy!

I like layering this particular flavor with Cinnamon-Apple Fridge Jam (page 256) or eating it with sliced apples.

DRAGON FRUIT AND WILD BLUEBERRY OVERNIGHT OATS

My hubby calls these my "designer" overnight oats because they have a beautiful marbled effect when layered in a glass jar. This recipe uses a couple of harder-to-find ingredients, but if you can track them down, it's a great flavor combination to try after you've been enjoying plain overnight oats for a while. Trader Joe's carries frozen wild blueberries, which happen to have considerably more phytochemicals and antioxidants than standard blueberries. I pair them with dragon fruit (also known as pitaya) because of its incredible color and unique mild, kiwi-and-pear-like flavor. Red dragon fruit is typically sold in small bags in the frozen fruit section of health food stores (fresh dragon fruit won't work for this recipe).

MAKES 2¾ CUPS (THREE SCANT 1-CUP SERVINGS)

1 (3.5-ounce) bag frozen red dragon fruit (see Note)
1 banana
¼ teaspoon vanilla powder or vanilla extract, or seeds from 1 vanilla bean (optional)
1 cup rolled oats
2 tablespoons plus 1 teaspoon chia seeds
1 cup unsweetened almond milk
1 tablespoon maple syrup
½ cup frozen wild blueberries

Fill a bowl with hot water and submerge the frozen dragon fruit packet for about 5 minutes to thaw.

Meanwhile, in a medium bowl, mash the banana with a fork or potato masher. Add the vanilla (if using) and combine well. Add the oats, 2 tablespoons of the chia seeds, and the almond milk and mix well. Set aside.

Once the dragon fruit is thawed, remove the packet from the water and drain the bowl. Empty the dragon fruit into the bowl, add the maple syrup and remaining 1 teaspoon chia seeds, and mix well. Add the blueberries (no need to thaw these) and combine well.

Divide the oat mixture among glass jars and top with the dragon fruit mixture. (For individual portions, I like using three widemouthed ½-pint jars, adding just under 1 cup of the oat mixture to each jar and topping each with ¼ cup of the dragon fruit mixture. Or I'll make a double batch and use 1-pint jars.) Seal the jars and refrigerate for at least 6 hours or preferably overnight before eating.

Storage: Store in the fridge in a glass food storage container or glass jars with tight-fitting lids for 5 to 7 days.

PLANT-POWERED MAYO SALADS

These are healthier iterations of beloved American fare—with chickpeas subbing in for tuna and tofu in place of egg—allowing you to enjoy these classic comfort foods while also reaping the unique health benefits of legumes and avoiding the more harmful cholesterol and saturated fats found in animal products.

You can use your favorite egg-based mayo, a store-bought vegan version, or my Cleanest Mayo (page 192). Just note that egg-based mayo will shorten the salad's shelf life.

CLASSIC CHICKPEA SALAD

When I was young, in the summer months, my mom would drop me off at my grandma's house for the day while she went to work. Luckily, my mom worked very nearby, so in the afternoon she'd come over and we'd all watch Grandma's favorite soap opera, *The Young and the Restless*, while enjoying a homemade lunch together. Loaded tuna salad sandwiches were a regular feature of those lazy summer lunches. My grandma was ahead of her time, always eating whole wheat bread and adding lots of fresh veggies and sometimes even apples and grapes to her tuna sandwiches. This is a classic vegan alternative to that dish, loaded with crunchy fresh veggies to nourish you and help fill you up!

MAKES 1½ CUPS (SIX ½-CUP SERVINGS)

1 (15.5-ounce) can chickpeas, drained and rinsed
¼ cup mayo, homemade (page 192) or store-bought
1½ teaspoons unsweetened plant milk
1 teaspoon Dijon mustard, or more to taste
2 tablespoons minced red onion
2 tablespoons grated carrot
2 tablespoons diced celery (stalk and leaves)
½ teaspoon dried dill
¼ to ½ teaspoon celery seed
Salt and ground black pepper

In a medium bowl, mash the chickpeas with a fork or potato masher, leaving some bigger bits for texture. Add the mayo, plant milk, and mustard and mix well. Add the onion, carrot, celery, dill, and celery seed and season with salt and pepper to taste. Stir to combine well.

Storage: Store in the fridge in a glass food storage container or glass jar with a tight-fitting lid for 7 to 9 days (or 3 to 5 days, if made with egg-based mayo).

Enjoy!

Chickpea salad sort of includes its own dressing, and that's why I love adding it right on top of my daily salad when I want to make it a full meal. It's also featured in the Classic Chickpea Salad Jars (page 298). Another fun way to enjoy this salad is on romaine lettuce leaf "boats," topped with microgreens or sprouts and drizzled with Creamy Balsamic Dressing (page 171) or Lemon-Garlic Tahini Sauce (page 172). And nothing beats a chickpea salad sandwich on warm toasted bread! My hubby and I like to use Ezekiel brand sprouted English muffins for open-faced sandwiches; I top mine with fridge pickles (see page 198), and he likes to top his with pickled jalapeños.

Curried Chickpea Salad: Add ½ to 1 teaspoon curry powder, ¼ teaspoon ground turmeric, and 2 to 3 tablespoons chopped fresh cilantro.

Herbed Chickpea Salad: Add an additional 1 tablespoon mayo, ¼ cup chopped fresh parsley, and ¼ cup chopped fresh cilantro, and replace the dried dill with ¼ cup chopped fresh dill. Adjust the salt as necessary.

VEGAN EGG SALAD

This recipe is astonishingly like the egg salad I remember from my pre-vegan days, but features one of my all-time favorite ingredients—tofu! It's especially easy because it doesn't require any cooking. (See page 270 for more info on cooking with tofu.)

MAKES JUST OVER 2 CUPS (ABOUT FOUR ½-CUP SERVINGS)

¼ cup plus 1 tablespoon mayo, homemade (page 192) or store-bought
1½ teaspoons nutritional yeast
½ teaspoon Dijon mustard
¼ teaspoon ground turmeric
¼ teaspoon salt (see Note)
1 (16-ounce) block firm tofu, drained and pressed for 10 minutes (see page 270)
Ground black pepper
1 tablespoon chopped dried or fresh chives or dried green onion

In a medium bowl, whisk together the mayo, nutritional yeast, mustard, turmeric, and salt to combine well. Set aside.

Chop the pressed tofu into roughly ¼-inch-thick strips, then into small chunks (leave some bigger pieces for texture). Add the tofu to the bowl with the dressing and stir to combine well. Stir in the pepper and chives.

Taste the salad and adjust the seasoning if needed.

Storage: Store in the fridge in a glass food storage container or glass jar with a tight-fitting lid for 7 to 9 days (or 3 to 5 days, if made with egg-based mayo).

Enjoy!

My hubby really loves this salad as an open-faced sandwich or wrap for lunch. For wraps, we use sprouted whole wheat tortillas (I like Alvarado Street Bakery brand), with pickled jalapeños or savory red onion fridge pickles (see page 198) and a heaping handful of baby spinach or mixed baby greens.

Note: While I think this dish tastes perfectly delicious as is, many vegans swear by using black salt (also known as kala namak) in vegan egg salad because of its uniquely egglike sulfur taste. Just be aware that it has considerably less sodium than regular table salt, so you'll likely need to add at least 1 teaspoon; adjust the quantity to suit your taste.

CHIA PUDDING

Chia seeds are perfect for no-cook puddings because they absorb liquid and form a natural gel. These tiny, mild-flavored seeds are packed with the omega-3 fatty acid ALA (alpha-linolenic acid) and are rich in soluble fiber, calcium, magnesium, and iron. They're also a phenomenal source of protein and fiber, which makes these puddings great for breakfast, as a snack, or for dessert!

CLASSIC VANILLA CHIA PUDDING

MAKES 1 CUP (ONE 1-CUP OR TWO ½-CUP SERVINGS)

3 tablespoons chia seeds
¾ cup unsweetened vanilla almond milk (see Note)
1 tablespoon maple syrup (optional; see Note)

In a small bowl, whisk together the chia seeds, almond milk, and maple syrup. Pour the mixture into a glass food storage container or glass jar, seal with the lid, and refrigerate for at least 24 hours to set before eating (see Notes).

Storage: Store in the fridge in a glass food storage container or glass jar with a tight-fitting lid for 5 to 7 days. If you're going to batch prep these for the week, I recommend leaving some of them on the top shelf toward the back of your fridge, as this typically extends shelf life the most.

Chocolate Chia Pudding: Add 1 to 1½ tablespoons unsweetened cocoa powder and increase the maple syrup to 1½ tablespoons.

Golden Chai Chia Pudding: Add 1 teaspoon ground cinnamon, ¼ teaspoon ground ginger, ¼ teaspoon ground turmeric, ⅛ teaspoon ground cardamom, ⅛ teaspoon ground cloves, and ⅛ teaspoon orange zest (optional, but highly recommended), and increase the maple syrup to 1½ tablespoons. You can also substitute reduced-fat coconut milk for the almond milk, if you wish.

Enjoy!

I love this classic vanilla pudding unsweetened, topped with fresh berries or Fridge Jam (pages 253–258). You can even prep the pudding with the berries right in the jars; just note that the shelf life will then be dictated by the berries (whole blueberries hold up the longest and will not affect shelf life). My kids and hubby love the chocolate variation and top theirs with berries, coconut flakes, and/or mini chocolate chips right when they're ready to eat.

Notes:

- If you don't have vanilla almond milk on hand, you can add ¼ teaspoon vanilla powder or vanilla extract or the seeds from ½ vanilla bean to plain almond milk.
- I happen to love this recipe without any added sweetener at all. If you're trying to eat less sugar, I highly recommend giving this pudding a try without the maple syrup.
- When I have the time—and remember to do it—I like to go in and give the puddings a stir after their first hour or two in the fridge. This helps to evenly distribute the chia seeds and discourage clumping.

DECADENT TROPICAL COCONUT CHIA PUDDING

This recipe is more involved than the simple chia pudding on page 217, so I generally think of it as more of a special-occasion dish and often serve it as a dessert when I have friends or family over. It has amazing flavor, as well as a beautiful presentation. This pudding is also richer and sweeter than the classic vanilla version, so I reserve it for the occasional treat.

MAKES THREE ½-PINT JARS

For the Chia Pudding

3 tablespoons plus 1 teaspoon chia seeds (black or white)
1 cup canned reduced-fat coconut milk
½ to 1 tablespoon maple syrup (depending on how sweet you like it)

For the Pineapple Chia Jam

¾ cup canned crushed pineapple, including a little bit of the juice (no more than 1 tablespoon)
1½ teaspoons chia seeds (I prefer white for color but black tastes just as good)
¼ teaspoon lime zest (optional, but highly recommended for flavor)
Pinch of ground ginger (optional)
Tiny pinch of salt (optional)

For the Coconut Topping

6 tablespoons unsweetened shredded coconut
1 tablespoon maple syrup
1 to 2 teaspoons pitaya powder (see Notes)

¾ cup diced mango, kiwifruits, or other fresh tropical fruit, for topping (optional)

Make the chia pudding: In a medium bowl, whisk together all the ingredients for the pudding; transfer to a glass jar, seal with the lid, and set aside.

Make the jam: In a small bowl, stir together all the ingredients for the jam; transfer to a glass jar and seal with the lid.

Refrigerate the chia pudding and jam overnight to set (see Notes).

Just before serving the pudding, make the coconut topping: In a small bowl, combine all the ingredients for the topping.

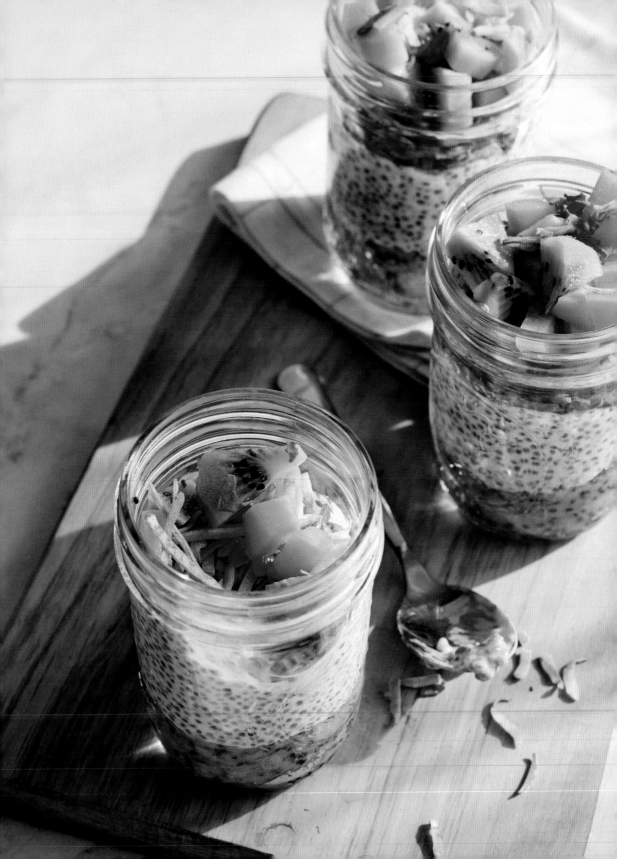

To assemble, spoon ¼ cup of the jam into each of three regular-mouth ½-pint glass jars. Add 6 tablespoons of the chia pudding to each jar. Top with ¼ cup of the diced fresh fruit (if using), then divide the coconut topping evenly among the jars and serve to excited *ooh*s and *aah*s!

Storage: Seal the jars with tight-fitting lids and store in the fridge for 3 to 5 days, depending on the diced fresh fruit used (mango keeps for at least 5 days); without the fresh fruit, they will keep for up to 7 days.

Notes:

- The pitaya powder is used to tint the coconut topping pink. I order pitaya powder online from Wilderness Poets; you might also find it in the baking aisle at Whole Foods (it's used as a natural food coloring for baking). If you can't find pitaya powder, you can use 1 teaspoon thawed frozen red dragon fruit instead; just note that the coconut will not be as crispy. Or you can skip tinting the coconut and get a pop of color by sprinkling fresh pomegranate seeds on top of the pudding instead.
- The coconut topping can be prepped ahead and stored in the fridge overnight as well but will lose its crispiness, so I prefer to make it just before serving.
- When I'm making this recipe as part of my weekly prepping instead of for a special occasion, I don't take the trouble to refrigerate the components individually before assembly. Instead, I prep the individual components, then layer them in the jars and refrigerate overnight to set before serving. While the presentation is a bit more rough and ready, the taste is still amazing!

FRIDGE BITES

You may know these as "bliss balls," but since they keep *forever* in the fridge, I've given them a little rebranding. I've cut down on the amount of nuts you'd typically see in these types of recipes and added oats for a bit of texture and crunch. I love that these are a completely self-serve snack and dessert option for the kids. They're great to bring along on road trips or family camping trips. The only problem in my household is portion control—you just want to keep popping these in your mouth!

Storage: It took me a while to actually get a gauge on shelf life because these would get eaten so quickly! But I'm happy to report that all three recipes keep in the fridge in a glass food storage container with a tight-fitting lid for 2 to 3 weeks.

CHOCOLATE BROWNIE FRIDGE BITES

MAKES 13 BALLS (ABOUT SEVEN 2-BALL SERVINGS)

½ cup raw walnuts
½ cup rolled oats
11 Medjool dates, pitted (about 1⅓ cups)
1 tablespoon maple syrup
¼ cup unsweetened cocoa powder
¼ teaspoon vanilla powder (or seeds from 1 vanilla pod or ¼ teaspoon extract)
Pinch of salt

Combine all the ingredients in a food processor. Process or pulse for 15 to 20 seconds, until the mixture comes together and forms a large ball of dough that travels around the bowl.

Use a cookie scoop to form the dough into 13 portions, placing them on a plate or parchment paper as you go, then roll each portion into a compact ball using your hands. The dough will be quite sticky (especially if you're using fresher dates), so it's a bit messy to work with. To help combat the stickiness, you can chill the dough in the fridge for a bit before forming the bites.

These can be eaten right away, but I recommend giving them at least a few hours in the fridge to firm up a bit first. Refrigerate in a single layer for at least 30 minutes to firm up before storing.

CARROT CAKE FRIDGE BITES

MAKES 14 BALLS (SEVEN 2-BALL SERVINGS)

1 cup rolled oats
1 teaspoon ground cinnamon
⅛ teaspoon ground nutmeg
⅛ teaspoon ground cloves or allspice
Pinch of ground ginger (optional)
Tiny pinch of salt (optional)
½ cup almond butter (see Notes)
½ cup golden raisins
1 tablespoon maple syrup
¼ cup shredded carrot

Combine the oats, cinnamon, nutmeg, cloves, ginger (if using), and salt (if using) in a food processor. Pulse for 1 or 2 seconds to distribute the spices throughout the oats. Add the almond butter, raisins, maple syrup, and carrot. Pulse for 10 to 15 seconds, until the mixture is crumbly and the carrots are well broken up.

Use a cookie scoop to form the dough into 14 portions, placing them on a plate or parchment paper as you go, then roll each portion into a compact ball using your hands.

Notes:

- Because these fridge bites use raisins instead of dates, the dough can be crumbly. This can be compounded if the nut butter you're using isn't as runny. I've found that sometimes I need to press the balls together in my palms rather than rolling them. I also recommend giving them a few hours in the fridge to firm up a bit before eating.
- One of the recipe testers for this book tried this recipe with sunflower butter and dates as substitutions because of allergies and reported that they were loved by her whole family.
- My hubby enjoys these best with the added pinch of salt to balance out the sweetness.

PEANUT BUTTER AND JELLY OATMEAL FRIDGE BITES

MAKES 14 BALLS (SEVEN 2-BALL SERVINGS)

1 cup rolled oats
½ cup salted creamy peanut butter (see Note)
½ cup golden raisins
1 tablespoon maple syrup
¼ cup dried cranberries

Combine the oatmeal, peanut butter, raisins, and maple syrup in a food processor. Process for 7 seconds just to combine. Scrape down the sides. Add the dried cranberries and pulse until they begin to break up a bit.

Use a cookie scoop to form the dough into 14 portions, placing them on a plate or parchment paper as you go, then roll each portion into a compact ball using your hands.

These can be eaten right away, but I recommend giving them at least a few hours in the fridge to firm up a bit first.

Note: You can substitute any other creamy nut butter you have on hand, though peanut butter is my favorite. If you don't have salted nut butter, just add a generous pinch of salt to the mix.

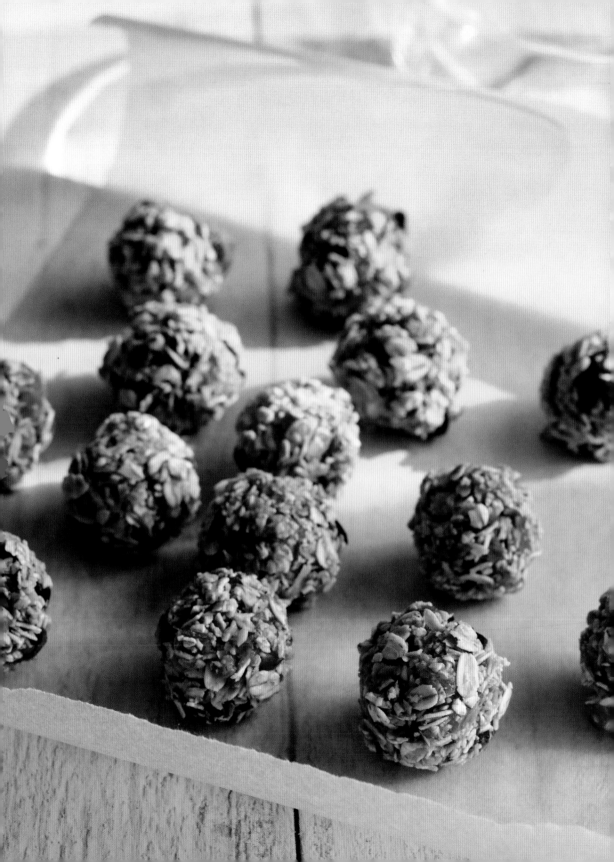

Cooked Prepping Recipes

One of the things I'm most proud of in my life has been developing my weekly prepping habit. Through my blog, I've passed this knowledge along, helping thousands of readers develop weekly batch cooking as the cornerstone to their pursuit of a Nutritarian lifestyle. Now, I'm so excited to give you a collection of plant-based recipes that will appeal to everyone, giving you incredible meal and flavor diversity, while also lasting you at least a week in the fridge!

PLANT-BASED SOUPS

I'm the one who's most likely to order a soup and salad at brunch. Yes, any time of the year—I'll eat soup indiscriminately on a 100-degree day just as I would on a 30-degree day. What makes soups so attractive from a health perspective is that simmering in liquid preserves more of the nutrients in the ingredients. They're also filling and naturally lower in calories than many other types of dishes.

But I'd argue the best part about soups, from a *prepping* perspective, is their incredible shelf life in the fridge and freezer! That's why I recommend making one or two batches of soup for the week as your first step into meal prepping.

Storage

- All the soup recipes in this book will keep in the fridge in a glass food storage container or glass jar with a tight-fitting lid for at least 9 days. Garden Veggie Minestrone Soup (page 228) and Chipotle Red Lentil Soup (page 230) will keep for up to 14 days.
- Most soups are great for freezing because their texture doesn't change as much as other cooked foods do. You can use glass jars for freezing soups; just make sure to leave at least 1 inch of headspace at the top in larger jars and at least ½ inch in smaller jars. Thaw overnight in the fridge before reheating. Thawed creamy soups should be whisked to reincorporate. I've also recently started using flexible silicone containers called Souper Cubes,

which are designed to store soups and sauces in ½- or 1-cup portions. Once the cubes are frozen, I transfer them to a silicone storage baggie. To reheat, simply drop one or two cubes into a pot and heat over medium-high.

Prepping Tips

- My favorite jars for soup storage are tall widemouthed 1-quart glass jars for multiple servings and widemouthed 1-pint jars for individual portions.
- To extend the shelf life of your soups, use a widemouthed funnel to transfer the soup to jars while it's still hot, then screw on two-piece metal lids. Combined with the residual heat of the soup, these lids form a kind of vacuum seal that maximizes freshness. Let cool and then store in the fridge. Just be careful when removing the lids later; they will be stuck on tight (I wear rubber gloves for protection). Note that this technique only works with mason jars and two-part metal lids, not other containers or lid types.

GARDEN VEGGIE MINESTRONE SOUP

Everyone should know how to make a great minestrone soup—it's such an easy and tasty way to eat lots of veggies!

MAKES 8 CUPS (ABOUT FIVE 1½-CUP SERVINGS)

½ tablespoon olive oil

½ medium yellow onion, diced

3 garlic cloves, pressed or minced

1 cup diced carrots

1 cup diced celery

½ teaspoon salt, plus more as needed

4 cups vegetable broth

1 cup diced tomatoes (preferably fresh)

1 (14-ounce) can kidney beans or great northern beans, drained and rinsed well

⅓ cup tomato paste

1 tablespoon no-salt seasoning (see page 159)

2 teaspoons dried oregano

1 bay leaf

½ zucchini, sliced

½ cup diced red bell pepper

½ cup water

¼ cup chopped fresh parsley

¼ cup chopped fresh basil

2 cups cooked pasta of your choice (see Note), preferably shells or elbows

Ground black pepper

In a large pot, heat the olive oil over medium-high heat. Add the onion and stir to coat with the oil, then cook until just beginning to color, 5 to 6 minutes. Add the garlic, carrots, celery, and salt and cook, stirring occasionally, for 5 to 6 minutes more.

Add the broth, diced tomatoes, beans, tomato paste, no-salt seasoning, oregano, and bay leaf. Stir to combine. Bring to a rolling boil, then reduce the heat to medium-low. Add the zucchini, bell pepper, and water and stir well to combine. Cook, stirring occasionally, for 20 minutes, then reduce the heat to low. Add the parsley, basil, and pasta and season with additional salt and pepper to taste. Simmer for 5 minutes more, then remove from the heat.

Serve immediately, or let cool completely before storing.

Storage: Store in the fridge in a glass food storage container or glass jar with a tight-fitting lid for up to 14 days.

Enjoy!

I love topping this soup with Classic Vegan Parmesan (page 190) and fresh herbs! I'll also sometimes put a heaping handful of fresh spinach in my bowl before ladling the hot soup on top.

Notes:

- Green lentil pasta and chickpea pasta do well in this soup. If you're having trouble finding bean pasta in one of the recommended shapes, it's fine to substitute whatever shape you can find. You could also use your favorite wheat- or rice-based pasta.
- Cook the pasta in a separate pot until al dente according to the package instructions, then drain before adding it to the soup.

CHIPOTLE RED LENTIL SOUP

This is my hubby's favorite soup, and it's based on a soup we had at a restaurant when we were celebrating our anniversary a few years back. I don't think more than two weeks have gone by where I haven't prepped this recipe since I first developed it. It has an incredibly delicious flavor that comes from cumin and chipotle peppers in adobo sauce. The lentils and quinoa combine to provide hearty flavor and a pleasing texture. If you're a fan of Mexican flavors, this is a must-make recipe.

MAKES 10 CUPS (FIVE 2-CUP SERVINGS)

½ medium yellow onion, diced
3 medium carrots, coarsely chopped
3 celery stalks, coarsely chopped
8 cups vegetable broth
1 cup dried red lentils
¼ cup uncooked tricolor quinoa
1 (14.5-ounce) can diced tomatoes
½ teaspoon ground cumin
1 (7-ounce) can chipotle peppers in adobo sauce (see Notes)
Salt and ground black pepper

In a large stockpot with a lid, cook the onion over medium-low heat, stirring occasionally, until translucent and lightly browned, 5 to 7 minutes. (By cooking over lower heat, you won't need to add any oil to the pot; the onions will gradually release moisture as they cook.) Add the carrots and celery and increase the heat to medium. Cover the pot with the lid and cook for 3 to 5 minutes, until the vegetables are just beginning to soften. Stir well.

Add the broth, lentils, quinoa, tomatoes, and cumin and stir well. Measure 3 tablespoons of the adobo sauce (or more, if you want a spicier soup) from the can of chipotles into the soup and stir well; reserve the chipotles and remaining adobo for another use (see Note). Cover the pot and cook for 20 minutes, stirring every 5 to 7 minutes. Reduce the heat to low and simmer, stirring occasionally, for 10 to 15 minutes more, then remove from the heat.

Serve immediately, or let cool completely before storing.

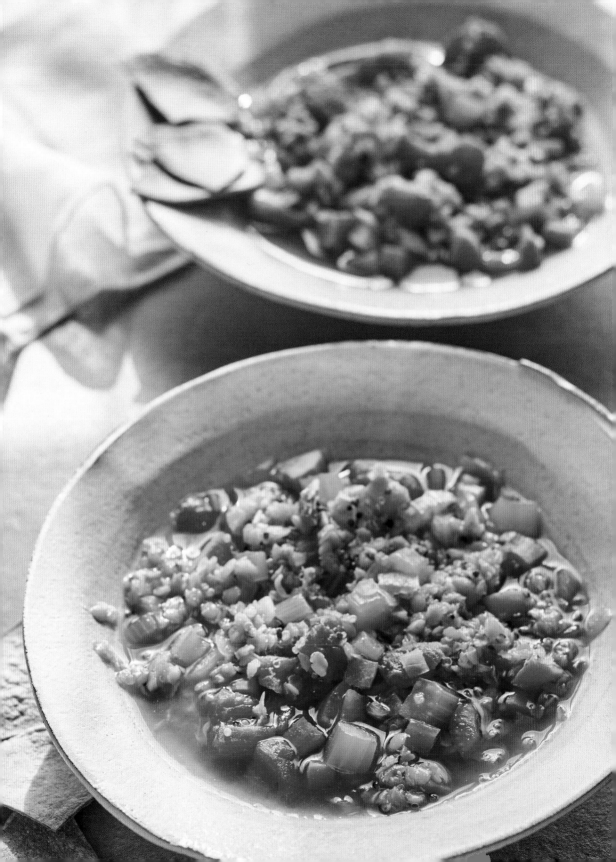

Storage: Store in the fridge in a glass food storage container or glass jar with a tight-fitting lid for up to 14 days.

Enjoy!

Serve with Oil-Free Tortilla Chips (recipe follows) and garnished with chopped fresh cilantro or Classic Vegan Parmesan (page 190).

Note: If you enjoy particularly spicy foods, you can dice one or two of the chipotle peppers and add them to the soup (my hubby prefers his this way). Transfer any remaining chipotles and adobo sauce to a glass jar with a tight-fitting lid and store in the fridge (preferably on an upper shelf near an airflow source) for up to 3 weeks. You'll typically have enough adobo sauce left over to make another batch of this soup. You can use the leftover chipotles to make Quick Pantry Salsa (page 194).

Oil-Free Tortilla Chips

Preheat the oven to 350°F. Line a baking sheet with a silicone baking mat or parchment paper. Cut four or five 6-inch corn tortillas into sixths or eight to ten 3½-inch corn tortillas into quarters. Arrange in a single layer on the prepared baking sheet. Bake for 25 to 30 minutes, until lightly browned all over, checking them halfway through baking. Let cool before serving.

COZY CORN CHOWDER

This recipe was inspired by my grandma Shirley's famous corn chowder. I felt like there was no place warmer, safer, and more perfect than Grandma's kitchen. My version subs out white potatoes for sweet potatoes and uses no oil or dairy. For a bit of protein and bite, garnish with edamame and sprinkle with Classic Vegan Parmesan (page 190).

MAKES 7¾ CUPS (SIX 1¼-CUP SERVINGS)

4 cups vegetable broth
1 small yellow onion, diced (1 cup)
3 medium celery stalks, diced (1 cup)
2 to 3 garlic cloves, minced or pressed (½ teaspoon)
2 medium sweet potatoes, cut into large dice (2 packed cups)
¼ teaspoon dried thyme
4 cups frozen or fresh corn kernels
¼ teaspoon salt
⅓ cup diced roasted red peppers (optional)

In a stockpot, heat ¼ cup of the broth over medium-high heat. Add the onion, celery, and garlic and cook until the onion is softened and translucent, 5 to 7 minutes.

Add the remaining 3¾ cups broth, the sweet potatoes, and the thyme and mix well. Raise the heat to high and bring the soup to a rolling boil (uncovered); this will take 8 to 10 minutes.

Add the corn and stir well. Reduce the heat to medium and cook for 15 minutes more, then remove from the heat.

Transfer just less than half the soup to a high-speed blender. (If you have a high-speed blender that has a hot soup setting, you can immediately pour the soup into the blender jar; otherwise, wait for the soup to cool before transferring it to the blender.) Blend until smooth and creamy, about 20 seconds, then return the blended soup to the pot and mix well. Taste the soup and season with salt. Stir in the roasted peppers (if using).

Serve immediately, or let cool completely before storing.

Storage: Store in the fridge in a glass food storage container or glass jar with a tight-fitting lid for up to 9 days.

CREAMY GINGER-MISO SOUP

I've always enjoyed the classic miso soup you get at sushi restaurants. But traditional versions are often made with bonito broth, so once I went vegan, I decided not to enjoy that soup anymore. I created this veggie-filled rendition that has all the comforting flavor with an amazingly creamy texture.

MAKES 8¾ CUPS (ABOUT FOUR 2-CUP SERVINGS)

2 cups sliced leeks (white parts only, from about 2 leeks)
4 cups coarsely chopped cauliflower florets (from about 1 head)
4 garlic cloves, chopped
6 cups vegetable broth
1 teaspoon onion powder
1½ tablespoons white miso paste
1 (2-inch) piece fresh ginger, peeled and coarsely chopped
1 teaspoon distilled white vinegar or rice vinegar
¼ cup raw sesame seeds
Salt (optional)

In a large stockpot, combine the leeks, cauliflower, garlic, broth, onion powder, miso, and ginger. Bring to a boil over medium-high heat. Reduce the heat to medium-low and cook until the cauliflower is fork-tender, about 10 minutes. Remove from the heat.

Transfer the soup to a high-speed blender. (If you have a high-speed blender that has a hot soup setting, you can immediately pour the soup into the blender jar; otherwise, wait for the soup to cool before transferring it to the blender.) Add the vinegar and sesame seeds and blend until smooth and creamy, about 60 seconds. (Depending on the size of your blender, you may need to blend in two batches. Alternatively, use an immersion blender to blend the soup directly in the pot.) Give it a quick taste and season with salt if needed.

Serve immediately, or let cool completely before storing.

Storage: Store in the fridge in a glass food storage container or glass jar with a tight-fitting lid for up to 9 days.

Enjoy!

Because this soup is so creamy, I love topping it with crunchy sliced green onions and both black sesame seeds (roasted) and white sesame seeds (raw).

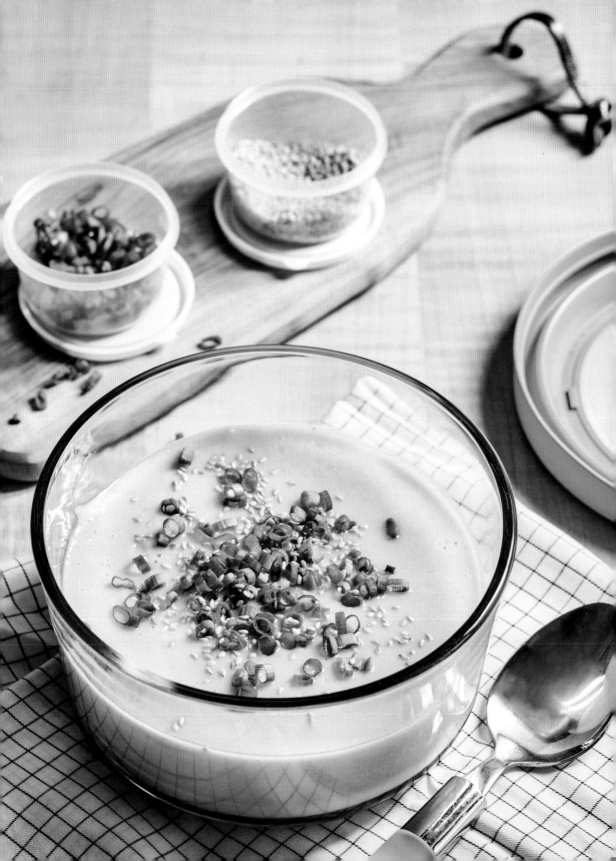

CREAMY MUSHROOM BARLEY SOUP

This recipe was inspired by several of my blog readers who told me they could drink my mushroom gravy like a soup. I use the same cauliflower cream sauce featured in that recipe, plus two of my favorite types of mushroom. The result is a creamy, decadent, flavorful, hearty soup that has quickly become one of my husband's most-requested vegan soups.

MAKES 6½ CUPS (ABOUT FOUR 1½-CUP OR FIVE 1¼-CUP SERVINGS)

½ large yellow onion, diced (1½ cups)

3 large garlic cloves, minced or pressed (1 teaspoon)

4 cups vegetable broth

5 ounces shiitake mushrooms, diced

8 ounces cremini (baby bella) mushrooms, stemmed (see Note) and sliced

1 teaspoon tamari

2 medium celery stalks, diced (½ cup)

2 medium carrots, diced (about ¾ cup)

½ cup pearl barley

1 teaspoon dried thyme

¼ teaspoon salt

Ground black pepper

1 cup Creamy White Sauce (page 240)

¼ cup diced roasted red pepper, drained and rinsed (optional)

In a stockpot, cook the onion over medium-high heat, stirring occasionally, until just softened, 5 minutes. Add the garlic and cook until a light brown crust forms on the pan (this makes things extra yummy), about another minute. Add ¼ cup of the broth and cook, stirring and scraping up the browned bits with a wooden spoon. Add the shiitake and cremini mushrooms and the tamari and cook for 5 minutes, then add the celery and carrots and cook for 5 minutes more.

Add the remaining 3¾ cups broth, the barley, thyme, salt, and pepper to taste and mix well. Increase the heat to high and bring the soup to a rolling boil (this will take about 10 minutes). Stir well, reduce the heat to maintain a simmer, and cook for 30 to 40 minutes more, until the soup has reduced by about half and the barley has softened and expanded.

Add the white sauce and mix well. Simmer for 5 minutes more, then remove from heat. Add the roasted peppers (if using) and mix well. If the barley has made the soup too thick for your liking, add some water to adjust the consistency.

Serve immediately, or let cool completely before storing.

Storage: Store in the fridge in a glass food storage container or glass jar with a tight-fitting lid for up to 9 days.

Enjoy!

I like to garnish this soup with chopped fresh parsley and Classic Vegan Parmesan (page 190). My hubby loves it with a salad for a stand-alone meal.

Note: Freeze the stems from the cremini mushrooms to use the next time you make Traditional Veggie Scrap Broth (page 314).

THAI CURRY BEET SOUP

I love taking different components I've already prepped for the week and turning them into something new. This adds variety to your meals and stretches out your preps. This simple-to-make dish turns two precooked components—roasted beets and caramelized onions—and a few pantry staples into a vibrant, flavorful soup!

MAKES ABOUT 5 CUPS (FOUR 1¼-CUP SERVINGS)

3 large beets (about 4 inches in diameter), roasted and chopped (see page 252)
½ cup No-Oil Caramelized Onions (page 250)
1 (13.5-ounce) can reduced-fat coconut milk
1 to 3 teaspoons Thai red curry paste (see Note)
½ cup water or Red Veggie Scrap Broth (see page 314)
Juice of ½ lime (sweet lime works the best; see Notes)

Combine all the ingredients in a high-speed blender. Blend on high for about 2 minutes, until smooth, creamy, and evenly colored (sometimes the coconut milk takes some time to blend in fully).

Transfer the soup to a pot and heat thoroughly before serving (or heat in the microwave). Or let cool completely before storing.

Storage: Store in the fridge in a glass food storage container or glass jar with a tight-fitting lid for up to 9 days.

Enjoy!

I like to garnish this soup with chopped beet greens and stems and/or Classic Roasted Chickpeas (page 279). The beet stems and leaves add a wonderful contrasting crunchy texture to the creamy soup, and the taste and added nutrition are amazing! I also love pairing this soup with Quick and Crispy Spinach and Artichoke Flatbreads (page 320) for a warming, filling, and beautiful lunch.

Notes:
- I recommend using Thai Kitchen brand curry paste. You can use green curry paste if you can't find red. You can increase or decrease the curry paste to your liking.
- I like this best with juice from a sweet lime, a variety of lime with less acidity than standard Persian limes. If you happen to find them at your supermarket, give them a try, but regular lime juice works fine, too.

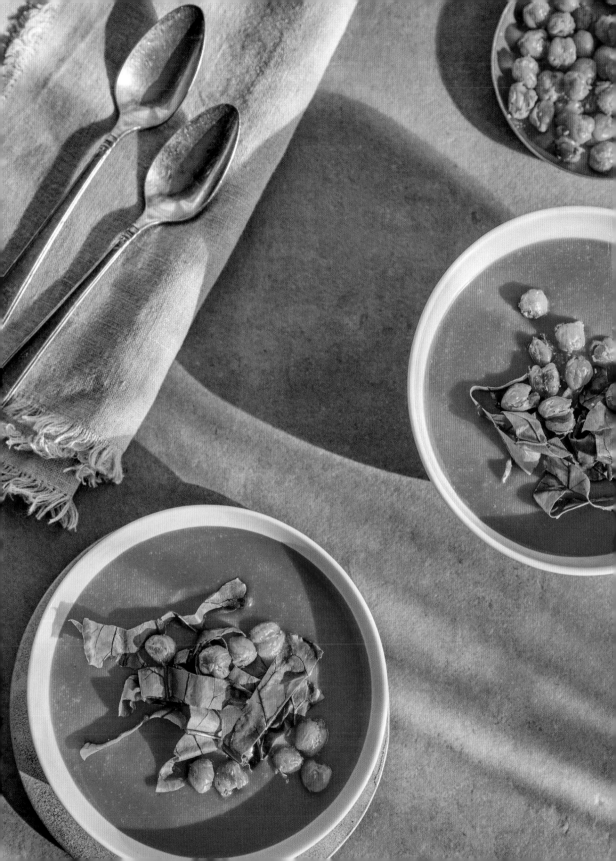

COOKED CONDIMENTS

I love fast, simple sauces the most, but in some cases, taking a bit longer to cook a sauce and develop its flavors is worth the extra time investment. These three cooked condiments are heavy hitters in elevating your meals and are well worth the extra effort.

CREAMY WHITE SAUCE

This sauce is my solution for adding creaminess without reaching for oil or dairy! I love that it has a couple of "hidden" veggies in there, too. It's used as a component in a couple of recipes here in this book, but don't be fooled—this sauce is a stand-alone star.

MAKES 2½ TO 3 CUPS (FIVE OR SIX ½-CUP SERVINGS)

½ head cauliflower, chopped into florets
½ small onion, diced into 1-inch pieces
⅓ cup plus 2 tablespoons raw cashews
1 garlic clove, peeled
¼ cup nutritional yeast
1 tablespoon liquid aminos
½ cup unsweetened almond milk

Place the cauliflower and onion in a stockpot and add water to cover. Cover the pot, bring to a boil, then uncover and cook until the cauliflower is just fork-tender, 4 to 5 minutes. Remove from the heat. Drain the veggies in a colander and let them cool just a bit.

Place the cashews in a high-speed blender and add the drained veggies. (The hot cooked veggies will help to soften the cashews.) Add the garlic, nutritional yeast, liquid aminos, and almond milk. Blend on high speed for about 60 seconds, until the sauce is smooth and creamy.

Storage: Store in the fridge in a glass jar with a tight-fitting lid for 9 to 12 days. Make sure to condense down your storage container throughout the week (see page 44). If you plan to keep this condiment for longer than 7 days, store it on an upper fridge shelf next to an airflow source.

Enjoy!

I love using this sauce as you would an Alfredo sauce, tossing it with al dente pasta or layering it with sliced veggies and noodles (I like green lentil noodles) for a creamy vegetable lasagna. This sauce makes a wonderful soup topper, too—try it with Garden Veggie Minestrone Soup (page 228). It's also used as a sauce for Dairy-Free and Still Delicious Creamy Mashed Potatoes (page 260) and in Creamy Mushroom Barley Soup (page 236).

SPINACH AND ARTICHOKE DIP

I love the challenge of taking a classic dish I used to love and crafting it so it can fit my healthy lifestyle while still providing me with that nostalgic flavor I crave! This dip really hits the spot for me—and even my hubby is smitten.

MAKES 2½ CUPS (FIVE ½-CUP SERVINGS)

1 (14-ounce) can artichoke hearts in brine (not oil), drained and rinsed

1 cup Cleanest Mayo (page 192)

1 tablespoon white miso paste

1 teaspoon lemon juice

¼ teaspoon onion powder

⅛ teaspoon cayenne pepper (optional)

Salt and ground black pepper

1 cup packed Simply Blanched Spinach (page 247), chopped (see Note)

⅓ cup No-Oil Caramelized Onions (page 250), chopped

½ to 1 cup Classic Vegan Parmesan (page 190) or panko bread crumbs, for topping

You can prep this dip ahead to bake later (or to use as a component in another recipe) or bake it to serve immediately. If you'll be serving the dip immediately, preheat the oven to 375°F.

Squeeze any remaining moisture from the artichoke hearts, then chop them and set aside.

In a medium bowl, combine the mayo, miso paste, lemon juice, onion powder, cayenne (if using), and black pepper to taste. Mix well, then taste and add salt if needed. Add the spinach, onions, and artichoke hearts. Mix very well.

If you'll be baking the dip later, transfer the mixture to a storage container or jar for storage (reserve the parmesan or panko separately). If baking the dip to serve immediately, transfer the mixture to a small baking dish and spread it evenly. Sprinkle with the parmesan or panko and bake until just beginning to brown, about 40 minutes.

Storage: Store in a glass food storage container or glass jar with a tight-fitting lid; uncooked, it will keep for 7 to 10 days, or 9 to 12 days cooked. Make sure to condense down your storage container throughout the week (see page 44). If you plan to keep this dip longer than 7 days, store it on an upper fridge shelf next to an airflow source.

Enjoy!

This dip is delicious fresh from the oven, served with Oil-Free Tortilla Chips (page 232) and crudités. But if you're prepping for later in the week, you don't need to bake the dip first—I like to keep it in a jar and then add it to bowls, soups, or salads. It's also a component in my Quick and Crispy Spinach and Artichoke Flatbreads (page 320).

Notes:
- This plant-based recipe doesn't have the same characteristic bubbly, cheesy texture as the traditional dip. For more cheesy flavor, feel free to add ½ to 1 cup of your favorite store-bought plant-based parmesan- or mozzarella-style cheese.
- You could substitute thawed frozen spinach if you don't have fresh; be sure to thoroughly squeeze out the excess moisture before using.

CREAMY MUSHROOM GRAVY

I initially created this decadent gravy for special occasions like Christmas and Thanksgiving to make my meal celebration-worthy. But my hubby and I love it so much that it's become a staple condiment in our fridge. It takes a bit more time than my other condiments, but the rich, decadent flavor is completely worth the extra effort.

MAKES 3½ CUPS (SEVEN ½-CUP SERVINGS)

1 ounce dried porcini mushrooms
5 cups water
¼ teaspoon salt
4 shallots, coarsely chopped
3 garlic cloves, coarsely chopped
1¾ cups vegetable broth, plus more if needed
1 tablespoon liquid aminos or tamari
1 tablespoon balsamic vinegar
2 teaspoons no-salt seasoning (see page 159)
2 teaspoons onion powder
¼ cup raw cashews
¼ cup raw pecans
¼ cup nutritional yeast
¼ teaspoon dried rosemary

In a saucepan, combine the dried mushrooms, water, and salt. Bring to a boil, then reduce the heat to medium-low and simmer until the liquid reduces by just more than half, 20 to 30 minutes. You should end up with 2 cups combined rehydrated mushrooms and concentrated mushroom broth. Remove from the heat and set aside. (This step can be done up to 4 days before you make the gravy. Just store the rehydrated mushrooms and their broth in the fridge in a 1-pint glass jar with a tight-fitting lid until you're ready to make the gravy.)

In a Dutch oven or large saucepan, combine the shallots, garlic, and ½ cup of the vegetable broth. Cook over medium-high heat for 10 to 12 minutes, until all the liquid has evaporated and a golden brown crust has formed on the bottom of the pan. Add the liquid aminos and stir, scraping up any browned bits with a wooden spoon.

Add ¼ cup more vegetable broth, then add the vinegar, no-salt seasoning, and onion powder. Cook for 7 to 10 minutes, until most or all the liquid is gone. Add the rehydrated mushrooms and their broth and mix well. Cook for 5 to 7 minutes more, until the whole mixture is bubbling hot. Remove from the heat.

Combine the cashews and pecans in a high-speed blender, then add the mushroom mixture. (If your blender has a hot soup setting, you can add the hot mixture right away; otherwise, allow it to cool slightly, about 10 minutes, before transferring it to the blender.) Add the nutritional yeast, rosemary, and remaining 1 cup vegetable broth. Blend on high until smooth and creamy, about 60 seconds. Adjust the consistency with more vegetable broth, if needed.

Serve immediately or let cool completely before storing.

Storage: Store in the fridge in a glass food storage container or 1-quart widemouthed glass jar with a tight-fitting lid for 12 to 14 days. Remember to condense down your storage container (see page 44) as you use the gravy.

Enjoy!

This is an incredibly tasty and earthy sauce that works for your 4-Step Preps (page 280) and is also used as a component in Comfort Prep Bowls (page 287). I love adding this sauce to lightly steamed greens and especially love it on fresh green beans. I'll also mix this gravy with a bit of Creamy White Sauce (page 240) and toss it with pasta as a kind of mushroom stroganoff.

MUST-KNOW COOKED VEGGIES

This collection of easy cooked veggies is inspired by my mother-in-law, Soo. In Korean cuisine, meals are always served with a selection of different cooked and pickled veggies that you can add to your dish as you like. These are the veggies I love to have stocked in my fridge during the week.

SIMPLE SAUTÉED GREENS

Fresh dark leafy greens can take up a lot of space in the fridge. Cooking them ahead of time frees up space and makes your life easier during the week. This simple and ultra-healthy method retains all the amazing nutrients found in greens, too!

MAKES 4¼ CUPS (ABOUT EIGHT ½-CUP SERVINGS)

¼ cup vegetable broth
5 cups packed stemmed curly kale or Swiss chard leaves, and/or baby spinach (see Note)
⅛ to ¼ teaspoon salt
Ground black pepper (optional)
1 teaspoon no-salt seasoning (see page 159; optional)

In a large pan or Dutch oven, combine the broth and the greens. Cook over medium-high heat, stirring, until the leaves turn bright green and just begin to soften, 2 to 3 minutes. Remove from the heat and stir in the salt, pepper (if using), and no-salt seasoning (if using).

Storage: Store in the fridge in a glass food storage container or glass jar with a tight-fitting lid for 9 to 12 days. Make sure to condense down containers (see page 44) throughout the week.

Enjoy!

Used as a component in 4-Step Preps (page 280) and Sweet Potato and Kale Prep Bowls (page 283).

Notes:
You can use just one type of green for the whole batch or a mix.

If desired, you can add up to 1½ teaspoons olive oil at the end of cooking, after removing the greens from the heat.

SIMPLY BLANCHED SPINACH

MAKES 1 TO 1½ PACKED CUPS (FOUR TO SIX ¼-CUP SERVINGS)

1 pound baby spinach
¼ teaspoon salt (see Note)

Bring a large stockpot of water to a boil. Separate the spinach into two batches. Plunge the first batch of spinach in the boiling water and cook for no more than 30 seconds; the leaves will wilt and turn bright green. Use a sieve to remove the spinach and immediately run it under cold water. Set aside. Repeat the process with the next batch; this time, you can drain the spinach in a colander since you're done with the cooking water. Let the blanched spinach stand until it's cool enough to handle, then use your hands to squeeze out excess moisture.

Place in a small bowl and add the salt. Serve immediately, or let cool completely before storing.

Storage: Store in the fridge in a glass food storage container or glass jar with a tight-fitting lid for up to 9 days. Make sure to condense down containers (see page 44) throughout the week.

Enjoy!

I use blanched spinach in Spinach and Artichoke Dip (page 242) and mixed with Korean Greens Sauce (page 249) as a component in Un-Fried Rice Prep Bowls (page 284).

Note: If you'll be serving the spinach with Korean Greens Sauce (page 249), omit the salt.

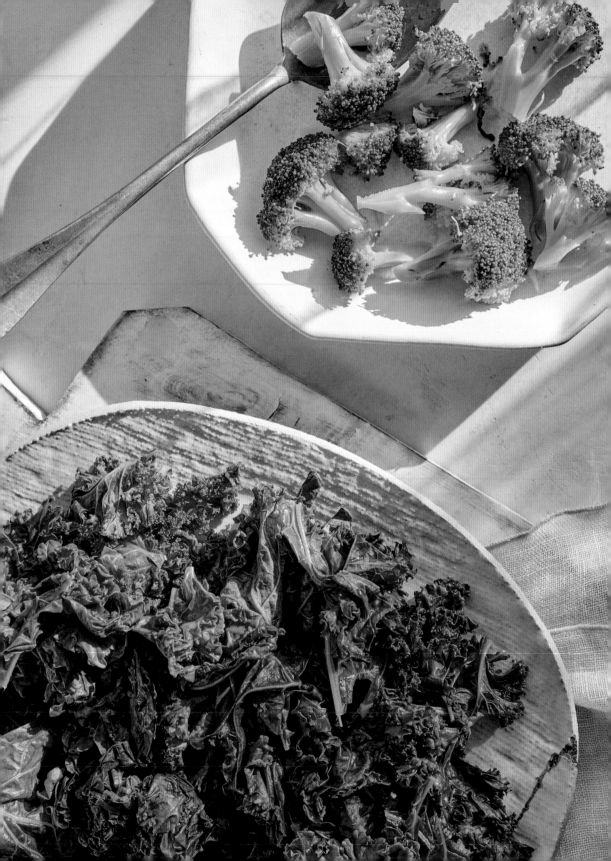

SIMPLY BLANCHED BROCCOLI

MAKES 4 CUPS (EIGHT ½-CUP SERVINGS)

4 cups broccoli florets
¼ teaspoon salt (see Note)

Bring a large stockpot of water to a boil. Add the broccoli and cook for no more than 1 to 2 minutes, depending on your preferred tenderness. You want the florets to stay crisp and bright green.

Drain in a colander and immediately run under cool water to stop the cooking, turning the florets with your hands to make sure they are all exposed to the water. (Alternatively, fill a large bowl with cold water and add the drained broccoli to stop the cooking.)

Storage: Store in the fridge in a glass food storage container or glass jar with a tight-fitting lid for up to 12 days. Make sure to condense down containers (see page 44) throughout the week.

Note: If you'll be serving the broccoli with Korean Greens Sauce (right), omit the salt.

KOREAN GREENS SAUCE

This flavorful, savory sauce is commonly used on banchan, small Korean side dishes served at family meals and restaurants. It works beautifully on blanched spinach or broccoli.

MAKES ABOUT ¼ CUP

2 tablespoons sliced green onions (white and light green parts only)
1½ tablespoons toasted sesame oil
1 teaspoon minced or pressed garlic
¼ teaspoon salt

Mix all the ingredients in small bowl. Use immediately or store.

Storage: Store in the fridge in a 4-ounce glass jar with a tight-fitting lid for up to 9 days.

Enjoy!

Toss with Simply Blanched Spinach (page 247). Or double the recipe and serve with Simply Blanched Broccoli (left).

NO-OIL CARAMELIZED ONIONS

These onions are easy to make, aromatic, savory, versatile, and hearty with rich onion flavor. I love having them on hand in the fridge to add to my daily salads, pile onto sandwiches, or use as a topper for my soup!

MAKES 1¼ TO 1½ CUPS (FIVE OR SIX ¼-CUP SERVINGS), DEPENDING ON ONION SIZE

2½ to 3 yellow onions (3 to 4 inches in diameter), sliced no thicker than ¼ inch
3 garlic cloves, minced or pressed
¼ teaspoon salt
2 tablespoons water

In a Dutch oven or other pan (see Note), cook the onions over medium-low heat for 10 minutes, stirring midway through. The onions will slowly release their moisture; around the 10-minute mark, you'll hear the sizzling start to increase and notice that moisture has been released. Add the garlic and salt and stir well. Cook for another 5 minutes.

Raise the heat to medium-high and cook until a golden brown crust forms on the bottom of your pan, 4 to 5 minutes. Add 2 tablespoons of water and stir well, scraping up any browned bits on the bottom of the pan. Cook for about 1 minute more, then reduce the heat to low and simmer the onions until all the moisture has been absorbed and they have a lovely caramel color, 5 to 7 minutes.

Storage: Store in the fridge in a glass food storage container or glass jar with a tight-fitting lid for up to 9 days. Make sure to condense down containers (see page 44) throughout the week.

Enjoy!

These are used as a component in Thai Curry Beet Soup (page 238) and Spinach and Artichoke Dip (page 242). My hubby also likes to add them to pita pizzas and baked potatoes.

Note: I recommend using an enameled cast-iron pan or Dutch oven or a stainless-steel pan. Nonstick pans don't allow the water to evaporate as well, so the onions get more steamed than caramelized.

THREE-INGREDIENT ROASTED MUSHROOMS

I live by a simple prepping motto: AHVR (Always Have Veggies Roasting). A big part of being a weekly prepper is getting efficient with your time in the kitchen, so you can get the maximum yield of different kinds of food in the same amount of time. When I'm making a soup, for example, I'll be sure to set something to roast in the oven first, since I'll be active in the kitchen during that time anyway. These mushrooms are almost always on the menu because they're so easy to make while being incredibly tasty for the effort.

MAKES ABOUT 1¼ CUPS (ABOUT FIVE ¼-CUP SERVINGS)

6 ounces mushrooms (white button, cremini/baby bella, or portobello varieties all work well)
1½ tablespoons coconut aminos
1 teaspoon no-salt seasoning (see page 159)

Preheat the oven to 375°F.

Quarter smaller mushrooms or slice portobello mushrooms. (I prefer to keep the stems on; if you don't, you can reserve them to use in Asian Veggie Scrap Broth, page 315.) Put the mushrooms in a glass baking dish. Sprinkle with the coconut aminos and no-salt seasoning and toss to coat.

Roast for 35 to 40 minutes. After the first 15 minutes, the mushrooms will begin to release their natural moisture; give them a good toss at this point. The mushrooms are ready when almost all of their moisture has been cooked out and their texture is still slightly soft. Remove from the oven and stir the mushrooms once more.

Serve hot, or allow them to cool completely before storing.

Storage: Store in the fridge in a glass food storage container or glass jar with a tight-fitting lid for up to 9 days. Make sure to condense down containers (see page 44) throughout the week.

Enjoy!

I add these to my Simple Rainbow Hummus Salad (page 178), serve them on top of soups, and use them in 4-Step Preps (page 280).

Note: If desired, after roasting you can add olive oil and/or salt to taste.

CLASSIC ROASTED BEETS

Because every home cook should know how to roast a beet! A couple of notes:

Beets come in a range of colors, but the most common varieties you'll find at supermarkets are red and golden. I like to buy fuchsia-fleshed red beets. You can identify these by looking at the stems. The more magenta-colored the stems, the more likely you'll have the same color flesh inside the roots.

I always try to find bunched beets with their beautiful leaves still intact. These are a two-for-one veggie because the stems and leaves are also delicious. I like to use the greens as I would salad greens and the stems as I would celery.

YIELD VARIES

Beets, loose or bunched

Preheat the oven to 375°F. Remove and store any beet stems and leaves. Scrub the beets well.

Wrap each beet in aluminum foil (smaller beets can be wrapped together in pairs) and place on a rimmed baking sheet or in a glass baking dish.

Roast smaller beets (3 inches in diameter or less) for 50 minutes and larger beets (4 to 6 inches in diameter) up to 1 hour 15 minutes. If you're not sure if they're done, poke them with a fork; they should be tender. Set the beets aside in the foil to cool; open the foil for faster cooling.

Once they are cool enough to handle, peel the skin off the beets using your thumb. You may need to cut off the top of the beet first to get it going. I like to cut roasted beets into large dice before storing.

Storage: Store in the fridge in a glass food storage container or glass jar with a tight-fitting lid for up to 12 days. Make sure to condense down containers (see page 44) throughout the week.

Enjoy!

I love adding these to my Simple Rainbow Hummus Salad (page 178) or eating them straight out of the oven tossed in Creamy Balsamic Dressing (page 171). These are also used in Beet Hummus (page 184), Beet-Berry Smoothies (page 208), and Thai Curry Beet Soup (page 238).

Note: I like to add beets to the oven when I'm baking other things to make the most of my time. They can cook at any oven temperature; just note that the lower the temperature, the longer the cooking time.

FRIDGE JAMS

Berries have a notoriously short shelf life, and sometimes you can get sour batches. One of my favorite ways to use up less-than-perfect berries is by making homemade fridge jam! (These recipes are called fridge jams because they're not canned for long-term storage, so they'll need to be stored in the fridge.) After doing this with my less-than-stellar berries for many years, I branched out to other kinds of fruit jams.

While the recipes on these pages include exact measurements, you can use this technique with whatever you happen to have on hand; general instructions follow. One other note: Be mindful that produce can vary widely, so cooking times for these fruit jams are approximate.

General Fridge Jam Technique

Step 1: Rinse your berries or fruit (if using frozen fruit, see Note). For apples, you can keep the skin on or peel them.

Step 2: Transfer the fruit to a pot. (The recipes that follow use a Dutch oven or other large pot, but use a smaller saucepan if you are making smaller batches.)

Step 3: Add a bit of citrus juice. This helps soften and break down the fruit and aids in preservation.

Step 4: Add a natural sweetener. My favorite way to sweeten these jams is with chopped pitted Medjool dates—the softer, the better. If you have harder dates, you can rehydrate with hot water in a small bowl for about 10 minutes before using. Using dates gives the jam more body and a thicker texture. The bits of dates will dissolve during cooking, but make sure to chop the dates into small enough pieces to facilitate cooking down. You can also sweeten with maple syrup; just note that the jam will not thicken as much.

Step 5: Bring the mixture to a rolling boil, then reduce the heat to maintain a simmer and cook until the fruit breaks down and the liquid condenses. Usually you don't need to add any extra water because the fruit releases moisture as it cooks down. If you have to add water, add no more than ⅓ cup at a time.

Step 6: Adjust the texture if needed. If you have too much remaining liquid or used maple syrup as your sweetener, you can add chia seeds to help thicken the jam. Remove from the heat and let cool before storing.

Storage: Because of the high sugar content in the dates, these jams enjoy a wonderful shelf life in the fridge! At a minimum, when stored in the fridge in a glass food storage container or glass jar with a tight-fitting lid, they will keep for 10 to 14 days and remain tasting super fresh; I've had batches stay fresh and delicious for almost 1 month.

Enjoy!

I use these fridge jams as components in Loaded Oatmeal Bowls (page 317) and Always Easy Parfaits (page 327); they are also great toppings for Classic Vanilla Chia Pudding (page 217) and Classic Vanilla Nice Cream (page 311).

Note: If you want to make these recipes with frozen fruit, I recommend allowing the fruit to fully thaw before making the jam. You will typically have more moisture with frozen fruit, so adjust accordingly. If using frozen berries, don't add any water to begin the recipe, only lemon juice; as the berries thaw, they will release liquid. Add water up to ⅓ cup at a time as needed as the jam cooks. You can also thaw frozen berries in a colander in the sink to drain excess moisture.

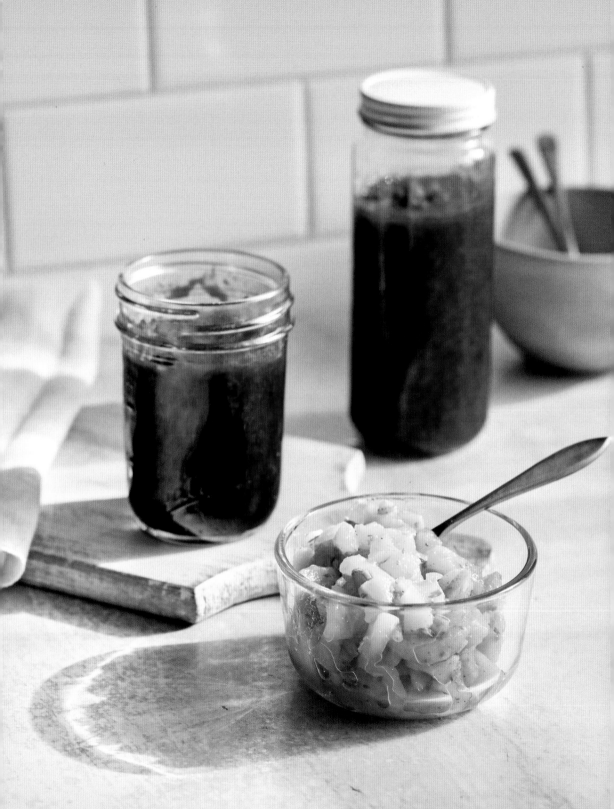

Clockwise from left: Blueberry, Raspberry, and Cinnamon-Apple Fridge Jams

CINNAMON-APPLE FRIDGE JAM

1⅔ cups water

2 tablespoons lemon juice (use only 1 tablespoon if you're using a tart apple variety)

8 apples (I love using the Opal variety because they break down easily)

8 Medjool dates, pitted and finely chopped

½ to 1 teaspoon ground cinnamon

Pour 1 cup of the water into a Dutch oven or other medium to large pot, add the lemon juice, and place the pot next to you as you prep the apples. Peel, core, and chop the apples into bite-size pieces, dropping them into the lemon water as you go; this will help prevent browning. Add the dates and the cinnamon and stir to incorporate.

Set the pot over medium-high heat and turn on your stove's exhaust fan to high (to help extract moisture as the apples cook down). Bring to the beginning of a rolling boil, stirring occasionally; this will take about 10 minutes. Stir well. Reduce the heat to low and add the remaining ⅔ cup water. Simmer for 20 to 30 minutes (depending on the texture of the apple variety), stirring every 5 to 6 minutes, until the fruit has cooked down and the liquid has evaporated.

Let cool completely before storing.

BLUEBERRY FRIDGE JAM

MAKES ABOUT 2 CUPS (FOUR ½-CUP SERV-
INGS)

18 ounces fresh blueberries
1 tablespoon lemon juice (or 1½ teaspoons if your dates are smaller or the
berries particularly tart)
5 Medjool dates, pitted and finely
chopped
¼ to ⅓ cup water, if needed

Rinse the blueberries well and put
them in a Dutch oven or other large
pot. Add the lemon juice and the
dates. Bring the mixture to the beginning of a rolling boil over medium-
high heat, stirring occasionally;
this will take about 10 minutes. The
blueberries will start to release liquid
and some will burst—this is what you
want to happen. You can add water
1 tablespoon at a time, if needed; you
want the texture to be beginning to
thicken.

Stir well and reduce the heat to
medium-low. Simmer the jam, stirring
every 5 to 7 minutes, until reduced
by half, 10 to 15 minutes. There will be
a few whole blueberries left.

Let cool completely before storing.

RASPBERRY FRIDGE JAM

MAKES JUST OVER 1½ CUPS (THREE ½-CUP OR
SIX ¼-CUP SERVINGS)

12 ounces fresh raspberries
1 teaspoon lemon juice
5 Medjool dates, pitted and finely
chopped (see Note)
2 tablespoons water, plus more if
needed

Rinse the raspberries well and place
them in a Dutch oven or other large
pot. Add the lemon juice and the
dates. Bring the mixture to the beginning of a rolling boil over medium-high
heat, stirring occasionally; this will
take about 10 minutes. The raspberries
will start to break down. You can add
water 1 tablespoon at a time, if needed;
you want the texture to be thick and
jamlike. The raspberries should all be
broken down at this point.

Stir well and reduce the heat to
medium-low. Simmer the jam, stirring
every 5 to 7 minutes, until reduced by
about a third, 10 to 15 minutes.

Let cool completely before storing.

Note: You can substitute 2 tablespoons
maple syrup for the dates. If using maple
syrup, pat your berries dry after rinsing
to remove excess moisture. You may also
need to thicken the jam with up to
1 tablespoon chia seeds, as the texture
will be a bit runnier without the dates.
The yield will stay roughly the same.

PEACH FRIDGE JAM

MAKES ABOUT 1¾ CUPS (SEVEN ¼-CUP SERVINGS)

4 large peaches, or just over 3 cups chopped frozen peaches
5 or 6 Medjool dates (depending on peach tartness), pitted and finely chopped
1 teaspoon lemon juice
1 cup water
¼ teaspoon ground cinnamon

Rinse the peaches, pit them, and chop them into small pieces. Put them in a Dutch oven or other large pot. Add the dates, lemon juice, and ½ cup of the water. Bring the mixture to the beginning of a rolling boil over medium-high heat, stirring occasionally; this will take about 10 minutes. Stir well and add the remaining ½ cup water. Reduce the heat to medium and cook for 5 minutes. The peaches should just be starting to break apart (depending on the variety and season, they may not break down much, and that's okay).

Reduce the heat to maintain a low simmer and cook the jam, stirring every 5 to 7 minutes, until reduced by about a third, about 20 minutes.

Let cool completely before storing.

ONE-POT MEALS AND SIDES

After soups, this recipe category is the perfect jumping-off point for getting into weekly meal prepping.

UN-FRIED RICE

This is one of the most well-reviewed recipes on my site—it's really amazing how much you don't miss the oil. While I never seemed to get full when eating takeout fried rice, this version leaves me totally satiated.

MAKES 4 CUPS WITHOUT TOFU (THREE 1⅓-CUP SERVINGS) OR ABOUT 5 CUPS WITH TOFU (FOUR 1⅓-CUP SERVINGS)

½ cup vegetable broth
¼ cup chopped green onions (white and light green parts only)
½ teaspoon minced or pressed garlic
½ cup diced red bell pepper
1½ cups thawed frozen vegetables (I like carrots and peas)
3 cups cooked brown rice (or substitute cooked quinoa or riced cauliflower)
1 to 2 tablespoons tamari
1 cup Tofu Eggs (page 274; optional)

Pour ¼ cup of the broth into a large skillet or Dutch oven. Add the green onions and cook over high heat for 5 minutes, or until the liquid has evaporated. Add the garlic and stir well.

Reduce the heat to medium-high and add the remaining ¼ cup broth and the bell pepper. Cook for 6 to 8 minutes, then add the thawed frozen vegetables and mix well. Cook, stirring, for 3 to 5 minutes. Add the rice and tamari; mix well. Add the tofu eggs (if using) and cook, stirring occasionally, for 5 minutes more, then remove from heat.

Storage: Store in the fridge in a glass food storage container or glass jar with a tight-fitting lid for up to 9 days. Make sure to condense down containers (see page 44) throughout the week.

Enjoy!

This is the main component in Un-Fried Rice Prep Bowls (page 284).

DAIRY-FREE AND STILL DELICIOUS CREAMY MASHED POTATOES

This is another of the most popular recipes from my site. Most of the nutrients in potatoes are found in their skins, so I leave them on for this recipe. They provide a great textural contrast to the creaminess. It's amazing how the creamy cauliflower-based sauce elevates these humble ingredients to rival any conventional mashed potatoes I've ever eaten.

MAKES ABOUT 6 CUPS (SIX 1-CUP SERVINGS), DEPENDING ON THE SIZE OF THE POTATOES

5 large russet potatoes
3 or 4 garlic cloves, smashed and peeled
¼ teaspoon salt
1½ cups Creamy White Sauce (page 240), or more as needed

Scrub the potatoes well, since you'll be leaving the skins on. Cut them into 1- to 1½-inch pieces and put them in a large stockpot. Add the garlic and water to cover, then add the salt. Cover and bring to a boil.

Remove the lid and cook until the potatoes are fork-tender, 5 to 7 minutes more, depending on the size of your potato chunks. Remove from the heat and drain. Return the potatoes and garlic to the pot and mash them—I like to leave a little bit of texture.

Add the white sauce and stir to combine; add more sauce if needed to achieve the desired consistency.

Storage: Store in the fridge in a glass food storage container or glass jar with a tight-fitting lid for up to 9 days. Make sure to condense down containers (see page 44) throughout the week.

Enjoy!

This is a great side dish anytime, but I also feature it in Comfort Prep Bowls (page 287).

QUINOA TABBOULEH

Quinoa is botanically related to nutritional powerhouses beets, chard, and spinach and is naturally gluten-free, low-glycemic, and nutrient-dense. But perhaps most important, it's delicious and extra-filling. Tabbouleh is a great use for this ancient grain, as the tasty oil-and-lemon-based dressing is the perfect complement to quinoa's nutty, subtle flavor.

MAKES 6 CUPS (SIX 1-CUP SERVINGS)

¼ cup lemon juice

¼ cup olive oil

3 garlic cloves, minced or pressed

1 teaspoon salt

Ground black pepper

3 cups cooked quinoa (I prefer white quinoa; see Notes)

1 large English cucumber, cut into ¼-inch slices, then quarter slices

4 Campari tomatoes, diced, or 1 cup diced fresh tomato of your choice

½ cup sliced green onions (white and light green parts only)

1 cup minced fresh curly parsley

¼ cup minced fresh mint

In a small bowl, whisk together the lemon juice, olive oil, garlic, salt, and pepper to taste; set aside.

Put the cooked quinoa in a large bowl. Add the cucumber, tomatoes, green onions, parsley, and mint to the bowl. Add the dressing and stir to mix well.

Storage: Store in the fridge in a glass food storage container or glass jar with a tight-fitting lid for 5 to 7 days. The veggies are crunchiest on the first day, but the flavor improves over the second and third days.

Enjoy!

I include this side dish in the Falafel Prep Bowls (page 288).

Notes:

- This recipe works best with chilled cooked quinoa.
- Many people find that quinoa has a bitter taste; this comes from a natural outer coating called saponin, which is an evolutionary defense against birds. A quick rinse under cool running water will ensure the best flavor.

EASY POTATO DAL CURRY

Whether you're working in an office or at home, this curry is easy to quickly heat up between meetings, making it a great lunch (or a great dinner). It's warm, comforting, and tasty, and a perfect prepping recipe for beginners since it's simple and keeps for a long time.

MAKES ABOUT 8 CUPS (FIVE 1½-CUP SERVINGS)

3 medium red potatoes
1 medium yellow onion, diced (about 1 cup)
3 garlic cloves, minced or pressed
2¼ teaspoons minced fresh ginger
1 (13.5-ounce) can reduced-fat coconut milk
1 cup dried golden lentils
2 cups vegetable broth
1 cup water, or more if needed
1 tablespoon curry powder
1 (14.5-ounce) can diced tomatoes, drained and rinsed well
1 cup loosely packed chopped stemmed Swiss chard leaves
Salt (optional)

Fill a large bowl with cool water. Peel the potatoes and cut them into large dice, placing them in the water as you go. Set aside.

In a large pot with a lid or Dutch oven, cook the onion over medium-low heat, stirring frequently, for about 7 minutes, until translucent and lightly browned. Add the garlic and ginger and cook, stirring, for 4 to 5 minutes, until just softening and fragrant.

Increase the heat to medium and add the coconut milk, lentils, broth, water, and curry powder. Drain the potatoes and add them to the pot as well. Cover and cook for 15 minutes, stirring once midway through.

Uncover, reduce the heat to medium-low, and stir well. Continue to cook for 15 to 20 minutes more, until the lentils have plumped and softened and the potatoes are fork-tender. You may need to add more water as the lentils and potatoes soak up the liquid.

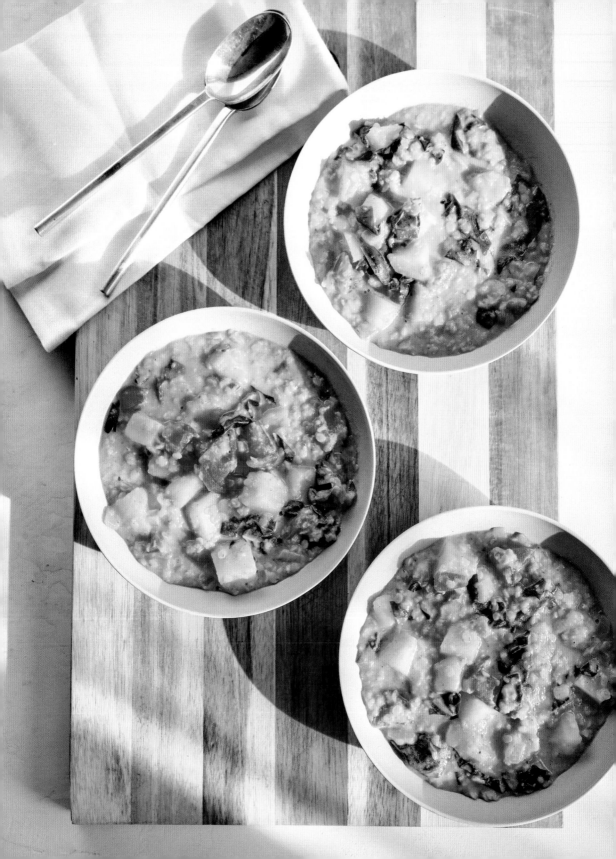

Add the tomatoes and mix well. Cook for 1 to 2 minutes more to heat them through, then remove from the heat and stir in the chard. Taste the dish and add salt if needed.

Storage: Store individual 1½-cup portions in 2-cup glass snap-lock storage containers or widemouthed 1-pint glass jars. Or store the full batch in a large glass food storage container with a tight-fitting lid. The dal will keep in the fridge for 9 to 12 days. This recipe also freezes well.

Enjoy!

This is a great stand-alone one-pot meal. Try adding ¼ to ½ cup cooked brown rice or quinoa (per portion) and/or topping with chopped fresh cilantro.

OIL-FREE FIRE-ROASTED SMOKY CHILI

Every home chef needs a hearty and satisfying chili recipe they love. This is one of my hubby's and my son's most-requested dishes. It's a vegan dish that's perfect for sharing with a crowd, as everyone can add their preferred toppings. This chili has a medium-hot heat level as written, with a smoky flavor and amazingly meatlike texture from the Tofu Taco Meat. If you have to make the Tofu Taco Meat, start it before the chili. After the tofu goes into the oven to bake, you can begin making the chili.

MAKES 7 CUPS (FOUR 1¾-CUP SERVINGS)

1 medium yellow onion, diced

3 garlic cloves, minced or pressed

2 tablespoons water

1 (12-ounce) jar roasted red peppers, drained, rinsed, and finely diced

1 (28-ounce) can fire-roasted diced tomatoes

7 ounces tomato paste

1 cup vegetable broth

1¼ teaspoons salt

2½ teaspoons ground cumin

1 teaspoon smoked paprika

1 teaspoon ground chipotle pepper (or your favorite chili powder; adjust quantity as needed for heat)

1½ teaspoons maple syrup

1 (15.5-ounce) can kidney beans, drained and rinsed

1 recipe Tofu Taco Meat (page 273)

In a large pot or Dutch oven, cook the onion over medium-low heat, stirring occasionally, for 7 to 10 minutes, until just softened. The onion will release its juices as it cooks down. Add the garlic and cook for 3 to 4 minutes, until a slight brown crust forms on the bottom of the pot. Add the water and stir, scraping up any browned bits from the bottom.

Add the roasted peppers, diced tomatoes, tomato paste, and broth and stir to mix well. Add the salt, cumin, paprika, chipotle, and maple syrup. Raise the heat to medium and bring the mixture just to a boil, about 10 minutes, then reduce the heat to maintain a simmer and add the beans.

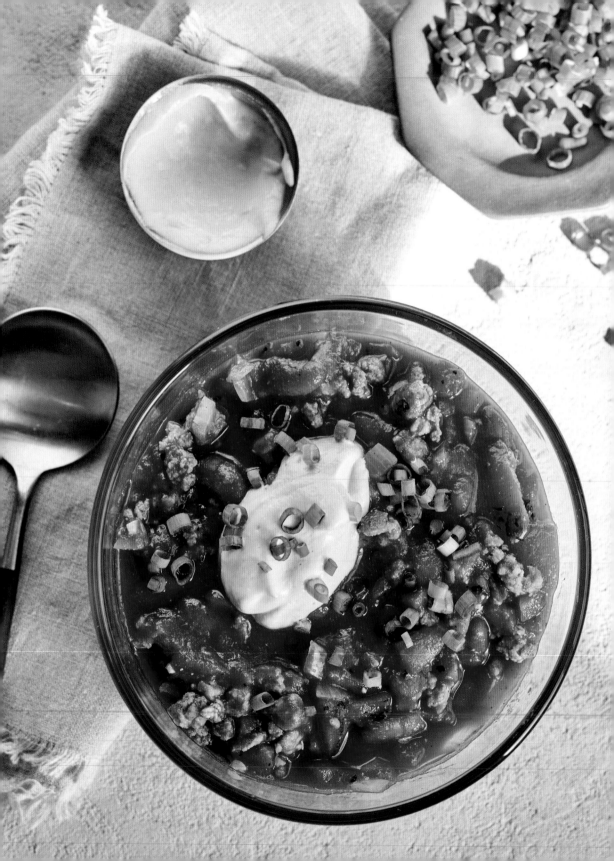

Cook for 15 minutes, then add the tofu taco meat. Reduce the heat to low and simmer, stirring occasionally, for 5 to 7 minutes, until the tofu has absorbed some of the liquid and softened a bit.

Storage: Store in the fridge in a large glass food storage container with a tight-fitting lid or portion individual servings into 2-cup glass food storage containers or glass jars with tight-fitting lids for 9 to 12 days. This recipe also freezes well for up to 2 months.

Enjoy!

You can add all sorts of toppings, such as cooked corn kernels, Creamy White Sauce (page 240), sour cream or yogurt (or nondairy versions), and sliced green onions or chives; serve with tortilla chips (such as Oil-Free Tortilla Chips, page 232) for dunking.

MEXICAN QUINOA CASSEROLE

There's nothing I love better than creating new ways to enjoy my favorite home-made cheese sauce! This recipe is another fine example of how you can create meal diversity using the components you prep for the week with a few common pantry and freezer staples.

MAKES 5 CUPS (FOUR 1¼-CUP SERVINGS)

1 cup jarred whole roasted red peppers (not packed in oil), drained and rinsed
3 cups cooked quinoa
1 cup cooked or canned black beans, drained and rinsed
1 cup thawed frozen corn kernels, drained
1½ cups Nacho Cheese Sauce (page 188)
¼ to ½ teaspoon ground chile (I use ¼ teaspoon chipotle powder)
5 tablespoons panko bread crumbs (optional)

Preheat the oven to 375°F.

Pat the peppers dry with a kitchen towel or napkins. Dice them and place in a large bowl. Add the quinoa, beans, corn, cheese sauce, and ground chile. Mix well.

If you are meal prepping, I recommend baking the casserole directly in individual containers; divide the mixture among four 2-cup oven-safe (such as tempered glass) food storage containers and set them on a rimmed baking sheet. If you will be serving it immediately, you can use a Dutch oven or small casserole dish instead. Sprinkle with the panko bread crumbs (if using).

Bake for 55 minutes, rotating the baking sheet or pot after 30 minutes. If serving right away, allow to rest for 5 minutes before serving. Otherwise, allow the containers to cool completely before storing.

Storage: Store in the fridge in individual glass food storage containers with tight-fitting lids (or in one larger container, if storing leftover casserole) for 7 to 9 days.

Enjoy!

Serve with your favorite salsa, Quick Pantry Salsa (page 194), Fresh Pico de Gallo (page 193), sliced avocado, and/or pickled red onion (see page 198). If you're meal prepping, store your garnishes separately to prevent the casserole from becoming soggy.

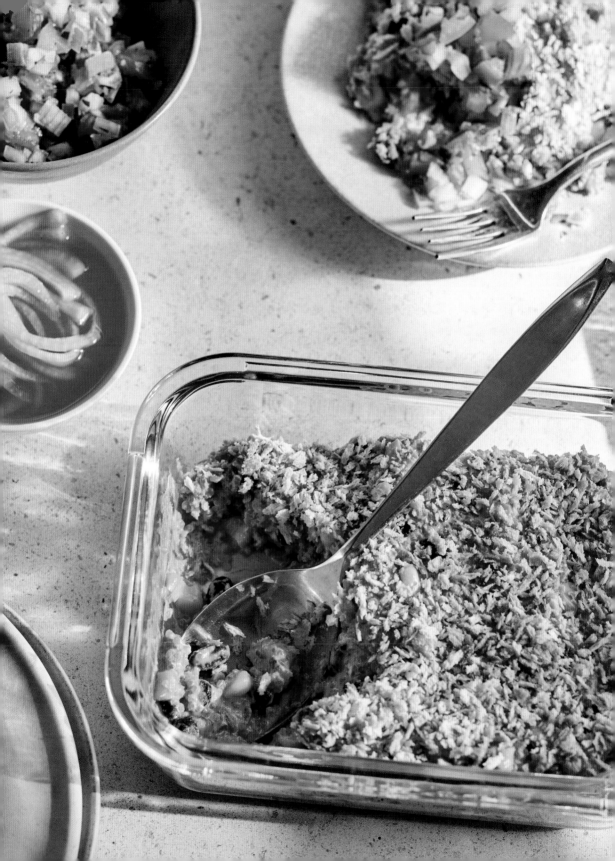

PLANT-BASED PROTEINS

Whatever your current dietary preference, these six recipes can have a place at your table! Whether you're looking to fully transition to a vegan lifestyle or simply add more plant-based dishes to your regular rotation, you'll find inspiration, simplicity, and amazing flavor in this recipe collection.

Tofu features prominently in this section: it's not tremendously processed, absorbs flavors easily, and is a family favorite in my house.

How to Press Tofu

To get maximum flavor and the right texture for your cooked tofu, you'll need to press the tofu before using it. This just means squeezing out as much water as possible. There are two ways to do this:

1. **DIY press:** Place the tofu on a plate or cutting board with a couple of napkins, paper towels, or cloth kitchen towels underneath and on top of the tofu block. Set a second cutting board or plate on top and add something heavy (I like to use cookbooks); and let the water press out.

2. **Store-bought tofu press:** I have two different tofu presses (both were gifted to me by my husband—likely as a bribe so I would make him more tofu recipes!). One of them is a stainless-steel model that holds one block of tofu. You place the press in the sink or over a plate to collect the liquid, then set the tofu block inside and place a very heavy weighted "lid" on top of the block. The second type is plastic and has space for two tofu blocks (which I love), as well as a built-in drip tray that collects the liquid. To use it, you place a block (or two) of tofu in the press, then screw down the two bolts that press the top plate against the tofu.

EASY BAKED TOFU

These chewy, savory, simple-to-make tofu strips are a great alternative to grilled chicken breast! My entire family loves these strips, and I'll often notice them disappearing as they cool while the kids just happen to walk ten laps through the kitchen. I love these fresh out of the oven, but they also keep well; I add them to salads, prep bowls, and sandwiches.

MAKES 24 STRIPS (SIX 4-STRIP SERVINGS)

2 (14- or 16-ounce) packages firm tofu, drained
⅓ cup coconut aminos
No-salt seasoning (see page 159)

Preheat the oven to 375°F. Line a baking sheet with parchment paper or a silicone baking mat.

Press the tofu for at least 10 minutes (see page 270). Cut each tofu block into 12 equal slices (about 1½ by 3½ inches). To do this I like to slice the block in half, then slice each half in half again—now you have fourths. Cut each fourth into 3 slices about ¼ inch thick.

Pour the coconut aminos into a small bowl or plate. Place one or two strips of tofu in the aminos for 1 to 2 seconds on each side, then transfer the coated strip(s) to the prepared baking sheet. Repeat to coat all the strips, then drizzle or brush any remaining coconut aminos evenly over the strips. Sprinkle liberally with no-salt seasoning.

Bake for about 50 minutes, until the strips are dry to the touch and the corners have lifted off the parchment. It's nice to rotate the pan at the 25-minute mark, but not essential. Check for doneness at the 40-minute mark; when you flip a strip over, it should be dry underneath with light speckling from the steam meeting the parchment. The texture will be a little crisp on the outside and chewy.

Storage: Store in the fridge in a glass food storage container with a tight-fitting lid for up to 10 days.

Enjoy!

These strips appear in Comfort Prep Bowls (page 287), as an optional protein source for the Colorful Lettuce Boats (page 181), and in Crunchy Thai Noodle Salad Jars (page 300).

Notes:

- If desired, you could use a salted seasoning blend or sprinkle on a bit of salt before baking. (The coconut aminos taste slightly sweet but are not overly salty.)
- One reader had a great cooking hack for this recipe: She places the strips in her panini press, where they cook in under 10 minutes!

TOFU TACO MEAT

One of my favorite meals growing up were turkey tacos, made from a boxed kit. My mom would use lean ground turkey and cook it in a skillet while I helped to remove and set up all the sauces and shells from the box. I set out to capture that nostalgic flavor and texture in this recipe—the result is even better than the real thing!

MAKES ABOUT 1¾ CUPS (ABOUT 3½ HALF-CUP SERVINGS)

1 (14- or 16-ounce) block extra-firm tofu, drained well
2 tablespoons reduced-sodium tamari
¼ teaspoon liquid smoke
2 teaspoons onion powder
1 teaspoon ground cumin
¼ teaspoon paprika
⅛ teaspoon garlic powder

Press the tofu for at least 30 minutes (see page 270)—you want it to be very dry.

Preheat the oven to 375°F. Line a baking sheet with parchment paper or a silicone baking mat.

Using your hands, crumble the pressed tofu into a medium bowl. You want a variety of sizes in the crumble; a combination of larger and smaller bits will add a variety of texture. Just be mindful not to overcrumble so you only have small bits left.

Add the tamari, liquid smoke, onion powder, cumin, paprika, and garlic powder to the crumbled tofu and stir and toss to incorporate well (take care not to crumble the tofu further as you mix).

Spread the tofu mixture evenly over the prepared baking sheet. Bake for 40 to 45 minutes, until golden brown, tossing the tofu once halfway through. It's okay for smaller bits to be more cooked or crispy while larger bits are softer.

Storage: Store in the fridge in a glass food storage container or glass jar with a tight-fitting lid for 10 to 12 days.

Enjoy!

Use as you would ground turkey. This is a main component in Oil-Free Fire-Roasted Smoky Chili (page 265), Taco Salad Jars (page 303), and Easy Taco Sliders (page 324). You can also add it to your favorite store-bought marinara to serve over pasta.

TOFU EGGS

As a toddler, my son loved scrambled eggs—then one day, he didn't. Recently he said he didn't like eggs anymore. But he loves these tofu eggs. Now my Saturday mornings as a short-order cook have gotten a bit easier! Sometimes you're *finally* ready for a change—if you're feeling like maybe you are, too, I think you're going to love this substitution.

MAKES 2 CUPS (FOUR ½-CUP SERVINGS)

1 (16-ounce) block firm tofu, drained
1 tablespoon vegetable broth
2 tablespoons nutritional yeast
¼ teaspoon ground turmeric
⅛ teaspoon garlic powder
Salt and ground black pepper

Press the tofu for at least 15 minutes (see page 270).

In a skillet or Dutch oven, heat the broth over medium heat. Crumble the pressed tofu into the pan with your hands. Cook, stirring frequently and breaking up the tofu with your spatula (you want a scrambled egg texture) for 5 to 7 minutes, until the moisture is gone.

Reduce the heat to low and add the nutritional yeast, turmeric, garlic powder, and salt and pepper to taste; stir to combine. Cook for another 5 to 7 minutes, until all moisture is absorbed, then remove from the heat.

Storage: Store in the fridge in a glass food storage container or glass jar with a tight-fitting lid for 10 to 12 days.

Enjoy!

These are a super-versatile scrambled egg substitute. They're used as an optional protein in Un-Fried Rice (page 259). Sometimes for Saturday brunch, my family makes easy breakfast tacos featuring this tofu plus fresh avocado, Fresh Pico de Gallo (page 193), pickled red onion (see page 198), and hot sauce or Quick Pantry Salsa (page 194). Other times we'll serve it with a toasted Ezekiel-brand English muffin topped with Classic Hummus (page 183) or mashed avocado sprinkled with no-salt seasoning. With some sliced Roma (plum) or heirloom tomatoes sprinkled with pepper, that meal will keep us going well into dinnertime.

TOFU MUSHROOM MEATBALLS

I always thought rolling individual meatballs was too labor-intensive for me, but using a cookie scoop to portion them out makes the process quicker. Plus, this recipe is irresistible! These meatballs pack a ton of meaty flavor while hiding the mushrooms enough to get past even the advanced radars of my mushroom-hating kiddos.

MAKES 26 MEATBALLS (FOUR 6-MEATBALL SERVINGS, PLUS A COUPLE TO SAMPLE OUT OF THE OVEN)

1 (14- or 16-ounce) block extra-firm tofu, drained
2 tablespoons tamari
8 ounces cremini (baby bella) mushrooms, stemmed (see Notes), caps coarsely chopped
½ small yellow onion (3-inch diameter), coarsely chopped
2 garlic cloves, pressed or minced
1 tablespoon flaxseed
¼ teaspoon liquid smoke
¼ teaspoon dried basil
1 cup panko bread crumbs (see Notes)
Ground black pepper
Salt (optional)
2 tablespoons olive oil or nonstick cooking spray (optional)

Press the tofu for at least 40 minutes (see page 270)—you want it to be as dry as possible. (If you're using a tofu press, you can decrease this time to 30 minutes.)

Preheat the oven to 375°F. Line a baking sheet with parchment paper or a silicone baking mat.

Using clean hands, roughly crumble the pressed tofu into a medium bowl (it's okay to have some bigger bits in there). Add the tamari and mix well. Transfer ½ cup of the tofu to a food processor and set the remainder aside.

Add the mushrooms, onion, garlic, flaxseed, liquid smoke, basil, and panko to the food processor. Season with pepper to taste. Process for no more than 10 seconds. You want a crumbly texture; bigger bits here and there are okay, but you don't want any extra-large chunks of onion.

Add the mushroom mixture and the salt (if using) to the bowl with the remaining crumbled tofu and mix together well with your hands or a spoon. The color of the mixture at this stage will be quite gray, with bits of white tofu showing through—don't be put off by this. The meatballs will have a lovely golden brown color after baking.

Use a 2-tablespoon (1-ounce) cookie scoop to portion the mixture, then roll each portion into a ball with your hands, placing them on the prepared baking sheet as you go. You can drizzle the meatballs with the oil or spray with cooking spray, or you can cook these without any oil—it's up to you!

Bake for 40 minutes, until golden brown, flipping the meatballs once halfway through.

Storage: Store in the fridge in a glass food storage container or glass jar with a tight-fitting lid for 10 to 12 days.

Enjoy!

These are the main protein component in Sweet-and-Sour Meatball Prep Bowls (page 290) and Spaghetti and Meatball Prep Bowls (page 292). One recipe tester, Amy, enjoyed these in a meatball sub with her favorite marinara and some Classic Vegan Parmesan (page 190). I also like mixing together Creamy White Sauce (page 240) and Creamy Mushroom Gravy (page 244) to make a sort of stroganoff sauce, serving it with these meatballs, a bed of pasta, plus Three-Ingredient Roasted Mushrooms (page 251) and Simply Blanched Broccoli (page 249).

Notes:
- Save the mushroom stems for Veggie Scrap Broth (page 312).
- To make these gluten-free, you can use almond meal instead of the panko bread crumbs. The texture will be slightly different, but they will still taste great.

BROCCOLI FALAFEL

I had so much fun developing this recipe, and now I finally feel like one of the "cool kids" who can make restaurant-caliber falafel (that just so happen to be loaded with tons of good-for-you broccoli)! These falafel have an incredibly flavorful, savory, fresh, herbal taste. It's another more time-intensive recipe, but the flavor is absolutely worth it. As one tester put it, "A recipe I will make again and again—easy to make, filling, and delicious!"

MAKES 21 PATTIES (FOUR 5-FALAFEL SERVINGS, WITH 1 EXTRA TO SAMPLE OUT OF THE PAN!)

2 cups coarsely chopped broccoli florets

1 cup coarsely chopped fresh cilantro (about ½ bunch)

1 cup coarsely chopped fresh flat-leaf parsley (about ½ bunch)

¾ cup dried chickpeas, soaked overnight and drained (see Notes)

4 garlic cloves, minced or pressed

¼ cup lemon juice

1 teaspoon coarse sea salt

1 teaspoon ground turmeric

1 teaspoon ground cumin

Ground black pepper

½ cup almond meal (see Note)

½ cup oat flour, plus more if needed

Vegetable or olive oil, for frying

Place the broccoli in a microwave-safe bowl, sprinkle lightly with no more than ½ tablespoon water, and cover with a microwave-safe plate or bowl. Microwave on high for 2 minutes, or until just lightly steamed and bright green. Drain off all excess water. Allow to cool, uncovered, for at least 5 minutes.

Put the fresh herbs in a food processor, then add the steamed broccoli, chickpeas, garlic, lemon juice, salt, turmeric, cumin, pepper, and almond meal. (I've found things process the best when added in this order.) Process for 7 to 10 seconds, then scrape down the sides to make sure everything is incorporated. Repeat, scraping down the sides as needed, until the mixture is crumbly and moist. The texture is like a mince, and if you press it with a fingertip, it should just hold the indention.

Transfer the mixture to a bowl and add the oat flour. Mix well. If you rinsed your herbs before adding them (that is, if they had any water clinging to them), you may need to add a bit more oat flour to tighten the mixture. Use a 2-tablespoon (1-ounce) cookie scoop to portion the mixture into balls, then flatten them into small patties about 1½ inches in diameter.

Fill a skillet (I like using a cast-iron skillet) with about ¼ inch of oil and heat over medium heat. Fry the falafel for about 2 minutes on each side, until crispy with a golden brown crust. Transfer to a paper towel–lined plate to drain excess oil.

Storage: Store in the fridge in a glass food storage container or glass jar with a tight-fitting lid for 10 to 12 days.

Enjoy!

It's really hard not to eat all of these fresh out of the pan—I'm constantly swatting my hubby's hand away as they cool! They are the main component in the Falafel Prep Bowls (page 288). I love them on salads and in wraps, too, or I'll serve them as an appetizer for family gatherings.

Notes:

- Make sure to use uncooked dried chickpeas—this gives the falafel the best mouthfeel and texture! Soak the dried chickpeas in water for 20 to 24 hours before making the recipe; they will soften and double in size. You'll end up with about 1½ cups of soaked chickpeas. Drain them before proceeding with the recipe.
- Depending on where you purchase, almond meal can be labeled as either "almond meal" or "almond flour." Avoid "fine" almond flour, which is pure white, and instead look for a product that includes visible brown bits of skin.

CLASSIC ROASTED CHICKPEAS

These roasted chickpeas are super simple, delicious, crunchy, flavorful, and satisfying. And the rather unfortunate news is that they're also incredibly addictive. Like, "sample while standing at the oven and before you've even realized it half the tray is gone" addictive!

MAKES 2 CUPS (FOUR ½-CUP SERVINGS)

2 (15-ounce) cans chickpeas, drained and rinsed
2 tablespoons olive oil
1 teaspoon salt

Preheat the oven to 400°F. Line a baking sheet with parchment paper or a silicone baking mat.

Lay the chickpeas out on a kitchen towel or several paper towels and pat dry. (It's okay if the skins come off; just discard them.) If you have a few minutes to let the beans continue to air-dry, this will help them get even crispier in the oven.

Transfer the beans to the prepared baking sheet and drizzle with the olive oil, stirring well to coat. Sprinkle with the salt and stir again.

Bake for 30 to 35 minutes, stirring and tossing once midway through the baking time, until the chickpeas are a light caramel brown color and all moisture has evaporated.

Serve immediately or let cool completely before storing.

Storage: Store in a glass food storage container or 1-pint glass jar with a tight-fitting lid. They will keep at room temperature for up to 24 hours or in the fridge for up to 9 days.

Enjoy!

My hubby and daughter love these as a snack. They also work wonderfully as a healthier crouton in salads and as a soy-free plant-based protein option in 4-Step Preps (page 280). These are a component in the Kale Caesar Salad Jars (page 297).

Note: Right out of the oven is when these will be the crispiest. After that, they will have a pleasing chewy texture.

4-STEP PREPS

Now we're at my favorite set of recipes. These delicious combos demonstrate how you can use the individual components elsewhere in this book to create hearty, well-rounded, make-ahead meals. I call them "prep bowls" because after reheating, you can easily arrange everything nicely in a bowl.

You can plug in the favorite recipes you discover in this book to create new meal combinations every week. The recipes in this section are six of my favorite combinations, but you can also create your own by following just four steps.

Step 1: Choose your base. These are the fiber-rich whole grains or veggies that will help form the foundation of your meal. My favorites include:
- Rice (brown, wild, cauliflower, or broccoli)
- Steamed or baked potatoes (colorful fingerlings or sweet)
- Quinoa
- Barley
- Amaranth (or other ancient grains)
- Pasta or noodles (I prefer whole-wheat or bean-based)
- Zucchini noodles

Step 2: Add cooked or raw veggies. I prefer green veggies because they're the most nutrient-dense, but you can switch things up for variety. They can be cooked or raw. I like lightly steamed veggies, so I'll often put raw veggies into my prepping containers so when I reheat them later, the veggies cook lightly but retain a still-crunchy texture. The sky is the limit in this category, but some of my favorite veggies are:
- Simple Sautéed Greens (page 246)
- Simply Blanched Spinach (page 247)
- No-Oil Caramelized Onions (page 250)
- Three-Ingredient Roasted Mushrooms (page 251)
- Classic Roasted Beets (page 252)
- Asparagus
- Brussels sprouts
- Green beans

- Carrots
- Cabbage

Step 3: Choose your protein. You can choose animal-based or plant-based protein options. My hubby and I often start with the same base preps and then add different proteins.

Plant-Based:
- Easy Baked Tofu (page 271)
- Tofu Taco Meat (page 273)
- Tofu Eggs (page 274)
- Tofu Mushroom Meatballs (page 275)
- Broccoli Falafel (page 277)
- Classic Roasted Chickpeas (page 279)

Animal-Based:
- Grilled or rotisserie chicken
- Cooked lean ground beef or turkey
- Hard-boiled eggs
- Meatballs
- Cooked lean sausage
- Grilled lean-cut beef

Step 4: Choose your sauce. There are abundant options to choose from throughout this book:
- Peanut Coconut Sauce (page 171)
- Tahini Yum Sauce (page 172)
- Creamy Balsamic Dressing (page 171)
- Lemon-Garlic Tahini Sauce (page 172)
- Golden Turmeric Sauce (page 173)
- Nacho Cheese Sauce (page 188)
- Sweet-and-Sour Sauce (page 191)
- Fresh Pico de Gallo (page 193)
- Quick Pantry Salsa (page 194)
- Vegan Ranch Dressing (page 195)

- Creamy White Sauce (page 240)
- Creamy Mushroom Gravy (page 244)
- Classic Hummus (page 183)
- Beet Hummus (page 184)
- Italian Herb Cannellini Bean Hummus (page 185)
- Your favorite marinara sauce
- Coconut aminos
- Tahini

Tip: You can turn any hummus into a sauce by thinning it out with water, or a combo of lemon juice and water, and adding a pinch of salt.

Bonus Step: Add condiments and toppings: These are the little extras that bring in color, contrasting flavor, and/or varying textures.

- Fridge Pickles (page 198)
- Classic Vegan Parmesan (page 190)
- Fridge Jams (page 253)
- No-salt seasonings (with seeds for crunch; see page 159)
- Raw nuts or seeds
- Fresh herbs

Storage: I like to use three-compartment glass food storage containers with snap-lock lids for these preps. Almost all of these recipes will keep in the fridge for at least 9 days (unless otherwise noted). Store portions you plan to eat later in the week closer to an airflow source. Please note that this shelf life only applies to the recipes as written. If you use animal products, the shelf life will decrease, so keep that in mind when meal planning. Many toppings and sauces are best stored separately from the other ingredients; I like to use reusable mini plastic containers that I found at the dollar store. Mine are 2⅜ inches wide and 1½ inches high and fit perfectly inside a three-compartment glass container.

Reheating: As a busy mom, I rely on reheating these prep bowls in the microwave. I cover the container with a microwave-safe plate (to prevent splatter) and microwave on high for 4 minutes. When I have more time to spare, I'll set the glass container (without its lid) on a baking sheet and reheat in a preheated 350°F oven for 6 to 10 minutes.

SWEET POTATO AND KALE PREP BOWLS

MAKES 4 PREP BOWLS

4 sweet potatoes
4 cups Simple Sautéed Greens (page 246, made with only curly kale)
Sauce of your choice (see Notes)

Preheat the oven to 400°F. Line a baking sheet with parchment paper or a silicone baking mat.

Wash the sweet potatoes well and pat dry. Pierce each potato several times with a fork. Place them on the prepared baking sheet and bake for 40 minutes to 1 hour, depending on their size, until fork-tender. Allow to cool completely.

Slice each sweet potato in half lengthwise and then cut them into 1-inch pieces. (Cutting and storing them this way helps when reheating the preps later.)

Portion the sweet potatoes and kale into four 3-compartment food storage containers or similar containers. Portion the sauce into small containers and add them to a compartment in the larger containers (if they fit) or store nearby in the fridge.

Storage: Store in the recommended containers in the fridge for up to 9 days. See page 282 for further storage guidelines.

Notes:
- Technically, this is a 3-step prep recipe, and I've done that on purpose. I wanted to give you one prep bowl that you could make no matter how hectic things get.
- I suggest Lemon-Garlic Tahini Sauce (page 172) or Peanut-Coconut Sauce (page 171), but any of the Quick-Mix Sauces on pages 169–173 would work.
- You can add a protein from the list on page 281 to this bowl if you'd like to make this a full meal. I especially love this combo with Classic Roasted Chickpeas (page 279).

UN-FRIED RICE PREP BOWLS

MAKES 4 PREP BOWLS

1 cup shredded red cabbage
1 recipe Savory Brine (page 201)
1 garlic clove, pressed or minced
¼ teaspoon raw sesame seeds (optional)
1 recipe Simply Blanched Spinach (page 247)
1 recipe Korean Greens Sauce (page 249)
1 recipe Un-Fried Rice (page 259, made with tofu)

In a small bowl, combine cabbage, brine, garlic, and sesame seeds; set aside. (You can do this up to a day before making the bowls.)

In a small bowl, mix together the spinach and Korean greens sauce.

Portion the un-fried rice, pickled cabbage, and spinach into four 3-compartment glass storage containers. If you don't have this particular kind of container, you can store the rice and spinach together and the pickled cabbage separately. Or, if you prefer to eat the spinach cold, store all three components separately.

Storage: Store the containers in the fridge for up to 9 days. See page 282 for storage guidelines.

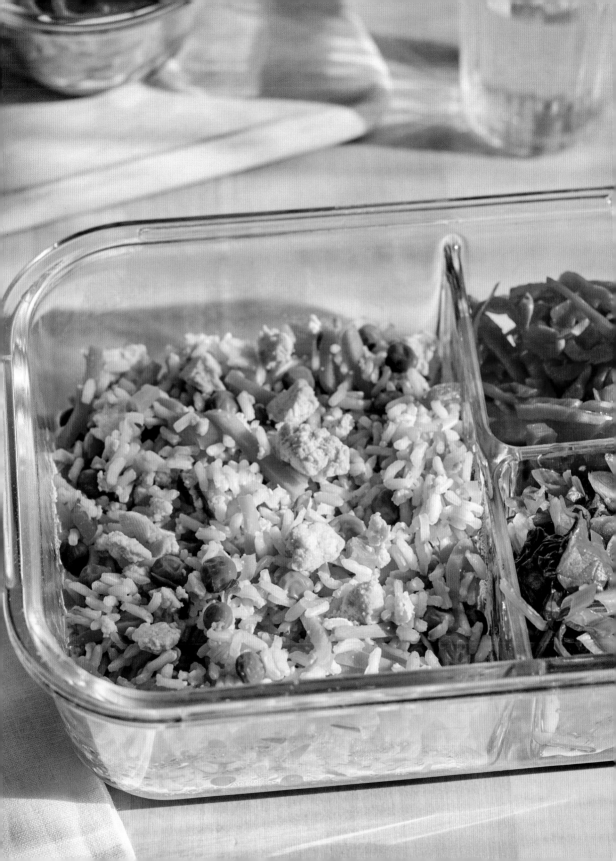

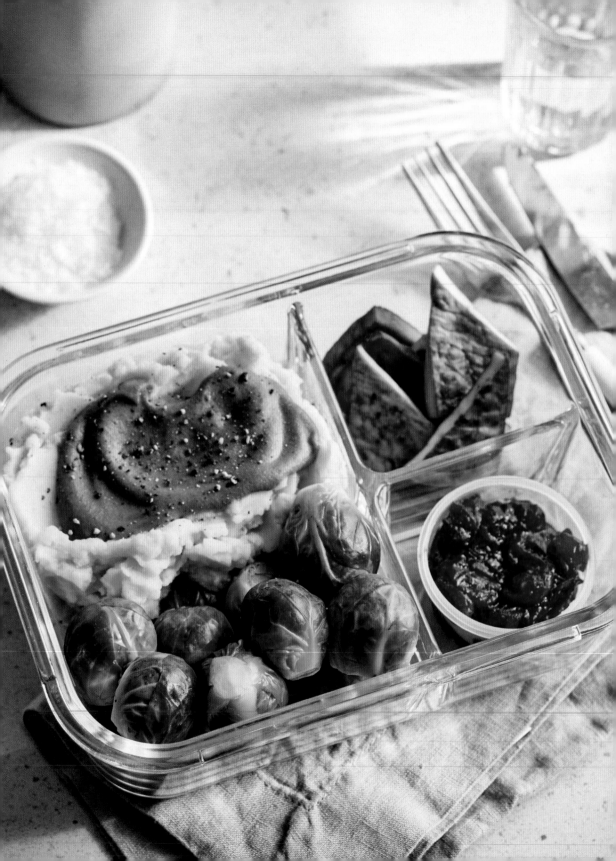

COMFORT PREP BOWLS

MAKES 4 PREP BOWLS

¼ cup water
1¼ cups fresh or frozen cranberries
1½ tablespoons maple syrup
14 ounces fresh Brussels sprouts
4 cups Dairy-Free and Still Delicious Creamy Mashed Potatoes (page 260)
1⅓ cups Creamy Mushroom Gravy (page 244)
16 strips Easy Baked Tofu (page 271), sliced on an angle into thirds

In a small saucepan, combine the water, cranberries, and maple syrup and stir well. Cook over medium-high heat, stirring frequently, for about 7 minutes, until the mixture has reduced by half. Set aside. (This makes ½ cup cranberry sauce; you'll use 2 tablespoons per prep bowl.)

Lightly steam the Brussels sprouts (see page 99) and divide them evenly among four 3-compartment glass storage containers or similar containers.

Divide the mashed potatoes, gravy, and tofu among the storage containers. Divide the cranberry sauce among four small plastic sauce containers and add them to a compartment in the larger containers (if they fit) so you can easily pull it out before reheating the prep bowls.

Storage: Store in the recommended containers in the fridge for up to 9 days. See page 282 for further storage guidelines.

Note: I like my Brussels sprouts very lightly steamed with plenty of crunch left, so sometimes I'll skip steaming them initially and put them in the bowls raw so they lightly steam when I reheat the whole bowl in the microwave later.

FALAFEL PREP BOWLS

MAKES 4 PREP BOWLS

20 pieces Broccoli Falafel (page 277)

4 cups Quinoa Tabbouleh (page 261)

1⅓ cups pickled red cabbage (see page 201, made with Savory Brine)

1 recipe Lemon-Garlic Tahini Sauce (page 172)

Cut the cooked falafel in half (this helps when reheating in the microwave). Divide the falafel, tabbouleh, and pickled cabbage evenly among four 3-compartment glass food storage containers or similar containers. Divide the tahini sauce into four small plastic sauce containers and add them to the compartment with the cabbage in the larger containers.

Storage: The storage life on this prep bowl is a bit less than the others because of the tabbouleh; store in the recommended containers in the fridge for 5 to 7 days.

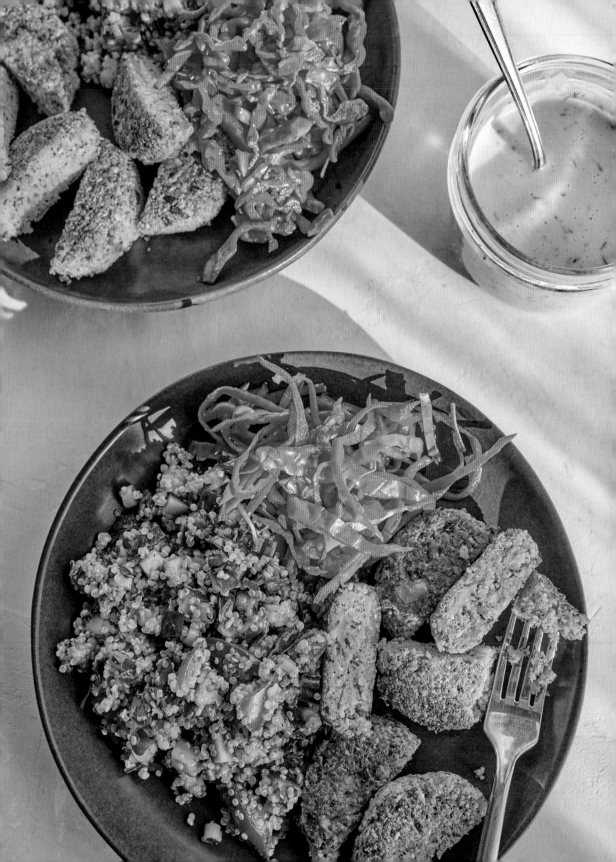

SWEET-AND-SOUR MEATBALL PREP BOWLS

MAKES 4 PREP BOWLS

½ tablespoon sesame oil

5 bell peppers (red, yellow, orange, or a mix), cut into large dice

1 cup chopped fresh or frozen pineapple

1½ teaspoons coconut aminos

1 recipe Sweet-and-Sour Sauce (page 191)

24 Tofu Mushroom Meatballs (page 275)

4 cups cooked brown rice or quinoa

In a pan or Dutch oven, heat the sesame oil over medium-high heat. Add the peppers and stir to coat well. Cook for 5 to 7 minutes, until the bottom of the pan is starting to brown. Add the pineapple and coconut aminos and stir well. Cook for 2 to 3 minutes, then reduce the heat to low.

Set aside 1 cup of the sweet-and-sour sauce; add the remaining ⅓ to ½ cup to the stir-fried peppers and pineapple. Mix well and remove from the heat.

Divide the meatballs, brown rice, and pepper-pineapple mixture among four 3-compartment glass food storage containers or similar containers. Portion the reserved sweet-and-sour sauce into four ¼-cup plastic sauce containers with lids (see Note). Allow everything to cool before storing.

Storage: Store in the recommended containers in the fridge for up to 9 days. See page 282 for further storage guidelines.

Note: I don't recommend storing the sauce directly on top of the other ingredients, as this causes the meatballs to get soggy. Instead, I store the sauce separately (either nestled inside the bigger containers or outside of them); when you're ready to reheat and eat, you can either add the sauce on top of the meatballs and rice before reheating, or heat everything separately and dunk and drizzle as you see fit!

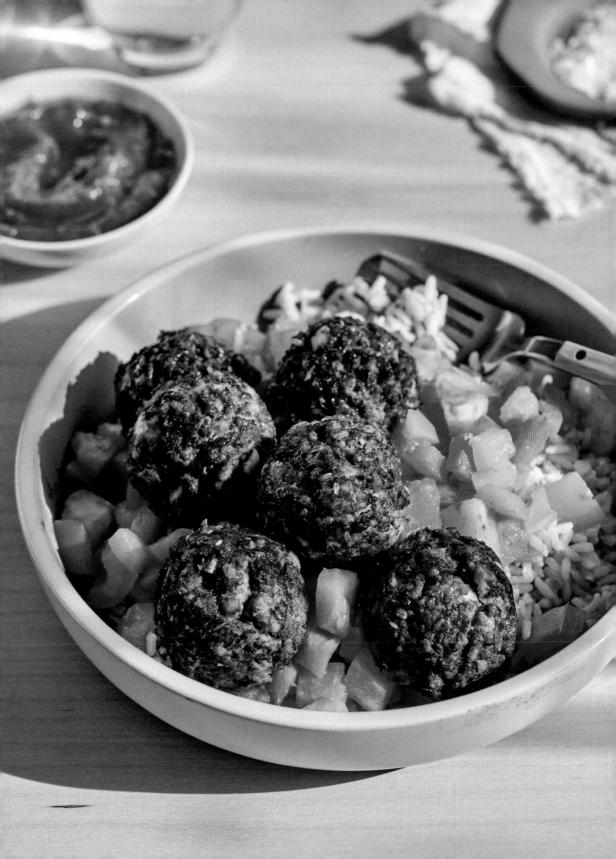

SPAGHETTI AND MEATBALL PREP BOWLS

MAKES 4 PREP BOWLS

24 Tofu Mushroom Meatballs (page 275), cooled completely
4 cups cooked spaghetti (I recommend bean-based or whole wheat)
2 cups of your favorite marinara sauce
1 recipe Simply Blanched Broccoli (page 249)
½ cup Classic Vegan Parmesan (page 190)

Divide the meatballs, spaghetti, marinara, and broccoli among four glass food storage containers (you can use 3-compartment containers or undivided ones). Portion the Parmesan into four small sauce containers and store separately.

Storage: Store in the recommended containers in the fridge for up to 9 days. See page 282 for further storage guidelines.

SALAD JAR PREPS

You can use the recipes in this group in two ways: prep them in jars, as written (handy for workplace lunches), or make them on demand.

The most important thing to remember when you're making a salad jar is to layer all the components in the jar from heaviest to lightest. In most of these recipes, I recommend storing the dressing separately in smaller containers. But you can also choose to add your dressing directly to the bottom of the jar; just make sure to layer the heartiest veggies (namely root veggies) in the bottom of the jar—they have to stand up to the moisture from the dressing.

To avoid condensation issues, it's best to start with cold ingredients—chill them in the fridge the day before you assemble your jars. If your fridge really struggles with condensation or it's particularly hot in your area during the warmer part of the year, chill the jars in the fridge overnight as well. This will create less work for your fridge and maintain the freshness longer.

My favorite way to eat a jar salad is by dumping it out into a bowl and mixing everything together. If you want to eat directly from the jar, you'll have to use jars that are larger than the salad itself (larger than what I've recommended in the recipes) so you have room to mix it up with your fork inside the jar. Note that storing your salad in larger jars will shave off some shelf life (1 to 2 days).

Storage: You can generally store your salad prep jars on any shelf in your fridge; place them toward the front of the shelf. If your fridge runs cold on the upper shelves, store the jars on a lower shelf. I like to store my salad jars in a row no more than two jars deep. (Remember, the freezing danger zone on certain fridge models is toward the back of your fridge, so be sure to leave 4 to 6 inches of space between the back wall and the jars—if you have a newer, higher-end model fridge, you don't need to worry about this as much.)

GREEK SALAD JARS

This is the perfect beginner-friendly salad jar prep recipe. It's a smaller side-salad size with an oil-based homemade vinaigrette, and you can store the dressing right in the jar!

MAKES 4 SALAD JARS

For the Greek Vinaigrette

¼ cup olive oil
3 tablespoons red wine vinegar
1 tablespoon maple syrup
2 garlic cloves, pressed or minced
¼ to ½ teaspoon dried oregano
¼ teaspoon salt
Ground black pepper

For the Salads

½ medium red onion, thinly sliced
1 cup whole cherry tomatoes
2 bell peppers (preferably green), diced
½ large English cucumber, sliced
¾ cup pitted whole black olives, or ½ cup sliced
4 cups baby spinach

Prepare the vinaigrette: In a small bowl, whisk together the olive oil, vinegar, and maple syrup. Add the garlic, oregano, salt, and pepper to taste. Whisk together well and set aside.

Assemble the salads: Divide the onion evenly among four widemouthed 1-pint glass jars. Add about 2 tablespoons of the vinaigrette to each jar to cover the onions. Then add the tomatoes, bell peppers, cucumber, olives, and spinach, dividing them evenly.

Top the jars with lids and store immediately in the fridge.

Storage: Store the jars in the fridge for 5 to 7 days. Note that the olive oil in the dressing may firm up a bit in the fridge but will be fine once tossed with the rest of the salad.

RAINBOW SALAD JARS

These jars just make me happy! Happy to see such a variety of good-for-me veggies and happy to be able to just reach into the fridge, grab my jar and a dressing, and be good to go. This makes a larger "main dish"-size salad, but you could scale down the quantities and use smaller jars, if desired.

MAKES 4 SALAD JARS

¾ cup diced yellow bell peppers
¾ cup shredded or diced carrots
¾ cup cherry tomatoes
¾ cup sliced red cabbage
1 cup diced green onions
6 to 8 cups chopped greens, such as romaine or loose-leaf lettuce, or whole baby spinach leaves
1 cup dressing of your choice (I like Vegan Ranch, page 195)

Divide all the toppings among four 24-ounce widemouthed glass jars (also called pint and a half jars) in this order: (1) bell peppers, (2) carrots, (3) cherry tomatoes, (4) red cabbage, (5) green onion. You'll have approximately 1 cup toppings total per jar.

Add 1½ to 2 cups of the greens, depending on how large a salad you prefer. You may need to really pack the greens in there.

Top the jars with lids and store immediately in the fridge.

Portion ¼-cup servings of the dressing into four sauce containers and store them close to the salad jars.

Storage: Store the jars in the fridge for 5 to 7 days.

Note: If you want to make this a heartier salad, you can add Easy Baked Tofu (page 271), Classic Roasted Chickpeas (page 279), or another protein of your choice just before serving (store these components separately).

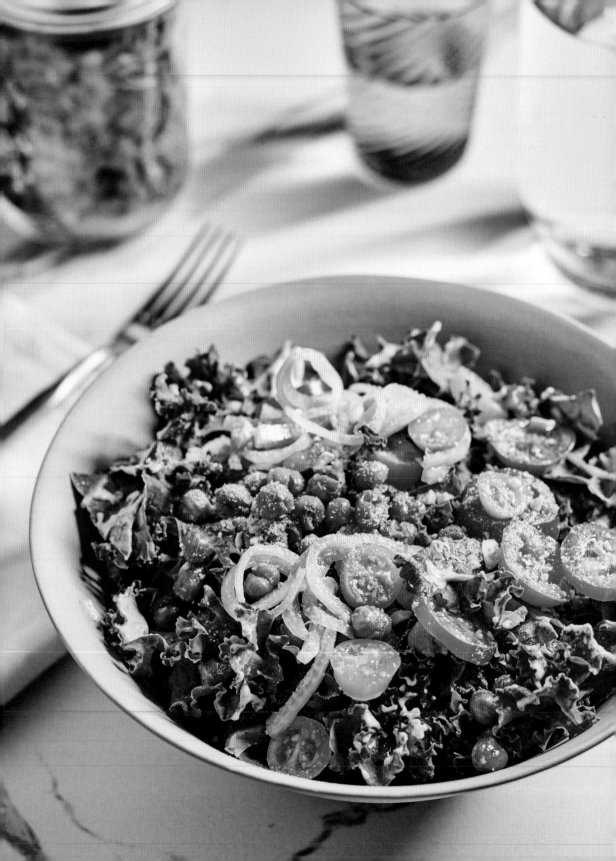

KALE CAESAR SALAD JARS

This is one of my favorite salad jar preps because it lasts so long in the fridge! Even though the shelf life below says 7 to 9 days, I have had jars stay fresh and taste amazing on days 10, 11, and 12! It's not surprising, since curly kale is one of the longest-lasting and sturdiest greens.

MAKES 4 SALAD JARS

1 recipe (2 cups) Classic Roasted Chickpeas (page 279)
8 cups chopped stemmed curly kale leaves
1 cup Cashew Caesar Dressing (page 196)
¼ to ½ cup Classic Vegan Parmesan (page 190)

Divide the chickpeas evenly among four widemouthed 24-ounce glass jars (also called "pint & half" jars; see Notes). Then add 2 cups of the kale to each jar, packing it in tightly. Portion ¼-cup servings of the dressing and 1 to 2 tablespoons of the parmesan into separate containers.

Storage: Store the jars in the fridge, with the dressing and parmesan stored separately, for 7 to 9 days (often longer).

Notes:
- I also like Weck brand 742½-liter Mold jars for these salads. Since these jars are slightly smaller, decrease the amount of kale to 6 cups (1½ cups per jar).
- You could make this salad anytime on demand instead of assembling the jars ahead. Use the individual portion sizes above for guidance. Put the kale in a bowl and add the dressing. Mix and massage well. Arrange on a plate or in a bowl and top with the chickpeas and parmesan. If I'm making this on demand, I like to add ¼ cup pickled red onions (see page 198) and sliced Roma (plum) or cherry tomatoes.

CLASSIC CHICKPEA SALAD JARS

MAKES 3 SALAD JARS

1 recipe (1½ cups) Classic Chickpea Salad (page 214)
3 cups packed baby spinach
¾ cup sliced red cabbage
1 cup grape tomatoes, or ¾ cup diced cucumber

Divide the chickpea salad evenly among three widemouthed 1-pint glass jars (see Note), then layer in the spinach, cabbage, and tomatoes or cucumbers. Top the jars with lids and store in the fridge immediately.

Storage: Store jars with cherry tomatoes in the fridge for 7 to 9 days; jars with cucumber will keep for 5 to 7 days.

Note: I also like Weck brand 742½-liter Mold jars for these salads. Since these jars are slightly larger, increase the amount of spinach to 4½ cups (1½ cups per jar).

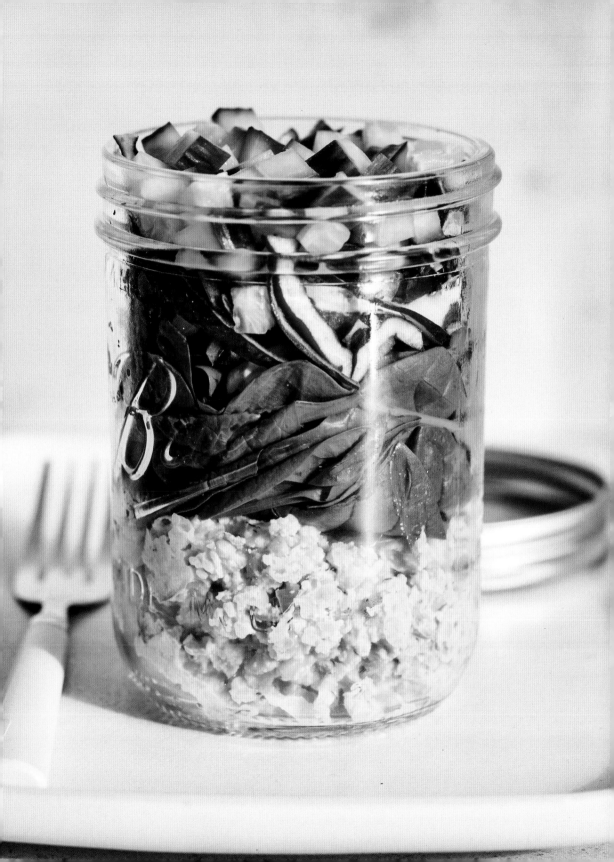

CRUNCHY THAI NOODLE SALAD JARS

MAKES 2 SALAD JARS

1½ cups cooked rice noodles
1 cup sliced red cabbage
⅔ cup sliced red bell pepper
⅔ cup grated carrots
½ cup thinly sliced cucumber or chopped sugar snap peas
½ cup diced green onions
1 cup fresh cilantro leaves
½ cup Peanut Coconut Sauce (page 171)
2 to 6 lime wedges, for topping (optional; see Note)
6 to 8 pieces Easy Baked Tofu (page 271), sliced, for topping (optional)
¼ cup crushed roasted peanuts, for garnish (optional)

Divide the rice noodles evenly between two widemouthed 24-ounce glass jars (also called "pint & half" jars). Layer in the cabbage, bell pepper, carrots, cucumber or sugar snap peas, green onions, and cilantro. Top the jars with lids and store in the fridge immediately.

Divide the sauce between two small storage containers. If using the lime wedges, tofu, and/or peanuts, divide them among separate individual containers. Store the sauce and toppings near the salads.

Storage: Store the jars in the fridge, with the sauce and toppings stored separately, for 7 to 9 days (often longer).

Note: I prefer to store the lime wedges separately and squeeze the juice over the salad just before serving. If you want to store them directly in the jars, arrange them cut-side down (skin up) on top of the cucumber or snap pea layer before adding the green onions and cilantro.

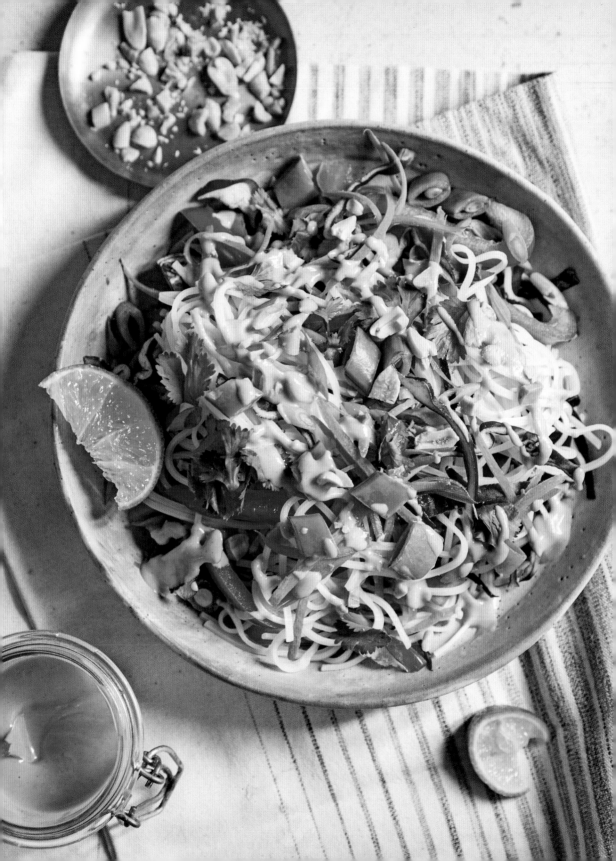

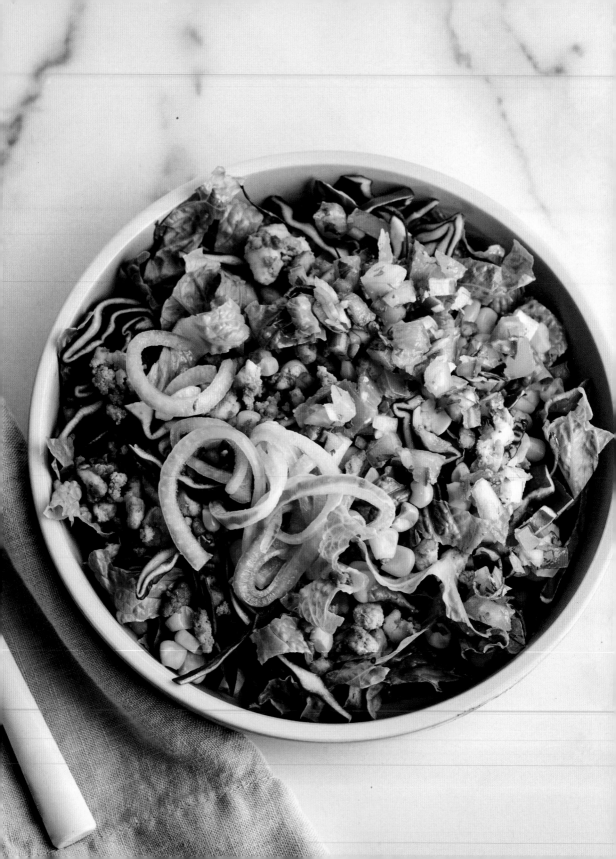

TACO SALAD JARS

MAKES 3 SALAD JARS

1½ cups frozen or fresh corn kernels

1 recipe Tofu Taco Meat (page 273), fully cooled

3 cups chopped romaine lettuce

¾ cup shredded or thinly sliced red cabbage

1½ cups Fresh Pico de Gallo (page 193) or your favorite salsa

1 cup pickled red onion (see page 198; optional)

Heat your corn kernels in the microwave until heated through, 2 to 3½ minutes. Let cool completely.

Divide the tofu taco meat evenly among three widemouthed 1-pint jars (see Note). Add ½ cup of the corn to each jar. Follow that with 1 cup of the lettuce (be sure to pack it in tightly) and ¼ cup of the cabbage.

Top the jars with lids and store in the fridge immediately.

Portion ½ cup of the pico de gallo and ⅓ cup of the pickled red onion (if using) into small storage containers and store them near the salads. (If you plan to eat the salads at home, it's fine to combine the salsa and pickled onion in the same container; if you're taking them on the go, it's best to use separate containers.)

Storage: Store the jars in the fridge, with the toppings stored separately, for 7 to 9 days (often longer).

Notes:
- I also like Weck brand 742½-liter Mold jars for these salads.
- When eating this salad, I like to empty the cabbage and romaine from the jar into my bowl first. I microwave the corn and taco meat directly in the jar for 2 minutes, then add them to the bowl and top with the pico de gallo and pickled onion.

Scratch-Made Extras

As I see it, a big part of the ecofriendly movement is regaining the knowledge and power to make things ourselves. Over the past few years, I've been inspired to find ways to reduce waste in my kitchen. This collection of easy DIY recipes will help you start to experiment with homemade versions of everyday items like plant milks and veggie broth, plus a few common household sweets that you can easily make using mostly bulk-bin ingredients. The more I make the effort to try my hand at things I'd otherwise buy, the more I realize how much better they taste and how rewarding it feels to do it myself!

PLANT MILKS

For the past four years, we've been a dairy-milk-free household! But even after we gave up cow's milk, I'd still cringe when I saw our recycling bin filled with almond milk cartons each week. I soon learned just how easy (and fun) it is to make your own plant milk. While we're not perfect in this practice, we've cut down our carton waste considerably over the past few years.

CLASSIC ALMOND MILK

Making homemade almond milk has become a bit of a family affair for me and my youngest. She enjoys the whole process, especially "milking" the almonds in the nut-milk bag and squeezing with all our might to get every last drop. When my family first tasted homemade almond milk, we realized just how bland the store-bought stuff really is. Do yourself a favor and give this simple recipe a try!

MAKES ABOUT 5 CUPS (FIVE 1-CUP SERVINGS)

1 cup raw almonds
4 cups water
¼ teaspoon vanilla powder or vanilla extract, or seeds from 1 vanilla bean (optional)
Pinch of salt
2 Medjool dates, pitted, or 1 tablespoon maple syrup (optional, for sweetened almond milk)

Place the almonds in a bowl and add cool water to cover. Set aside to soak for at least 8 hours and up to 24 hours (see Note). Drain the almonds and rinse well.

Put the almonds, water, vanilla (if using), and salt in a high-speed blender; add the dates if you'd like to sweeten the almond milk. Blend on high for 1½ minutes, or until creamy. (Blending for the full 1½ minutes will ensure you extract as much of the flavor and fats from the almonds as possible.)

Drape a smooth cotton kitchen towel (not terry cloth) or nut-milk bag over a large bowl or widemouthed 2-quart glass jar. Strain the almond mixture through the towel or bag, squeezing well to extract as much liquid as possible from the pulp. Reserve the almond pulp for another use or compost it.

Storage: Store the almond milk in the fridge in a glass beverage container or glass jar with a tight-fitting lid for up to 5 days. Natural separation will occur; just shake well before using. Almond pulp can be stored in the fridge in a glass food storage container or glass jar with a tight-fitting lid and little air exposure for 7 to 10 days.

Note: I've accidentally (many times) left my almonds to soak for longer than 24 hours. When I know I'm not going to get around to using them within 24 hours, I'll drain and rinse the almonds, return them to the bowl, and add fresh cool water to cover, then set them aside to continue to soak. I have used them at 48 hours and still gotten great results, but the shelf life does decrease by a couple of days. If you're in a pinch and don't have time for an 8-hour soak, you can soak the almonds in lightly salted hot water for an hour.

Pink Almond Milk: My daughter and I have made pink almond milk (use the sweetened version) by adding a few fresh strawberries and/or 2 teaspoons pitaya powder (see Note on page 221) before blending. Note that the shelf life will decrease to 3 days.

THREE-SEED CHOCOLATE MILK

3 cups water

4 Medjool dates, pitted, or 2 tablespoons maple syrup

⅓ cup hulled raw pumpkin seeds (pepitas)

⅓ cup hulled hemp seeds

2 to 4 tablespoons unsweetened cocoa or cacao powder

2 tablespoons ground flaxseeds

1 teaspoon vanilla extract (optional)

Pinch of salt

In a high-speed blender, combine the water, dates, pumpkin seeds, hemp seeds, 2 tablespoons of the cocoa powder, the flaxseeds, vanilla, and salt. Blend on high until very smooth and creamy. Taste and add more cocoa powder, if desired.

Serve chilled or heat in a small saucepan on the stovetop and serve as hot chocolate.

Storage: Store in the fridge in a glass jar with a tight-fitting lid for up to 5 days. (Not freezer-friendly.)

Note: This recipe is made for those with nut allergies. You could substitute other nuts or seeds in place of the pumpkin seeds or hemp seeds, but note that depending on the nuts used, you may need to strain the plant milk through a nut-milk bag after blending. Some nuts and seeds that would work well include cashews, almonds, pecans, walnuts, hazelnuts, pistachios, and hulled sunflower seeds.

PUMPKIN SPICE CASHEW CREAMER

MAKES 2½ CUPS (TEN ¼-CUP SERVINGS)

¼ cup raw cashews
2 Medjool dates, pitted, or 2 tablespoons maple syrup
2 cups boiling water
2 tablespoons canned pure pumpkin puree
1 teaspoon vanilla extract (optional)
1 teaspoon ground cinnamon
¼ teaspoon ground cloves
¼ teaspoon ground nutmeg
Pinch of ground ginger (optional)
Pinch of salt (optional)

Put the cashews and dates in a medium bowl and pour over in the boiling water (see Note). Set aside to soak for 15 minutes; do not drain.

Transfer the cashews, dates, and their soaking water to a high-speed blender. Add the pumpkin, vanilla (if using), cinnamon, cloves, nutmeg, ginger (if using), and salt (if using). Blend on high for 1 minute, or until very smooth and creamy. Add more water if desired to achieve your ideal consistency.

Storage: Store in the fridge in a glass jar with a tight-fitting lid for up to 5 days.

Enjoy!

Add 2 tablespoons of this creamer plus 2 tablespoons almond milk (such as Classic Almond Milk, page 304) to a mug of hot coffee in the morning. For iced coffee, add ¼ cup creamer and ½ cup almond milk to 1 cup chilled coffee.

Notes:

- This recipe calls for quickly soaking the cashews and dates, so you can put together this recipe in a hurry when you need your coffee in the morning but forgot you're out of creamer. If you plan ahead, you could soak them in room-temperature water overnight instead.
- If you're making Pumpkin Hummus (page 186), this creamer is a great way to use up some of the leftover canned pumpkin puree.

DIY STORE-BOUGHT SWEETS

OIL-FREE FRUIT-SWEETENED NUT OR SEED GRANOLA

This recipe is a family staple at my house. Because it's sweetened with fruit, it's a healthier alternative to store-bought granola (which often contains lots of sugar and oil); do note that it's not as sweet as commercial varieties. If you or someone in your family can't eat nuts, using tahini and sunflower seeds to make a nut-free version is equally delicious.

MAKES 5 TO 6 CUPS (SIX TO EIGHT ¾-CUP SERVINGS)

2 very ripe, spotty bananas
5 Medjool dates, pitted
¼ cup raw almond butter or tahini
1 teaspoon ground cinnamon
¼ teaspoon vanilla powder or vanilla extract, or seeds from ½ vanilla bean
3½ cups rolled oats
½ cup chopped raw walnuts or hulled raw sunflower seeds
½ cup golden raisins

Preheat the oven to 325°F. Line a baking sheet with parchment paper or a silicone baking mat.

Combine the bananas, dates, almond butter, cinnamon, and vanilla in a high-speed blender. Blend on high until smooth and creamy.

In large bowl, combine the oats and walnuts. Pour the banana-date mixture into the bowl (make sure to scrape down the sides of the blender jar) and mix well.

Spread the mixture evenly over the prepared baking sheet (clumps are okay and, in my opinion, preferred). Bake for 25 minutes, then remove the baking sheet and mix the granola well, breaking up any very large clumps. Bake for 20 to 30 minutes more, until the granola is dark golden brown. Let cool completely, then mix in the raisins.

Storage: Store at room temperature in a glass food storage container or glass jar with a tight-fitting lid for up to 14 days.

Enjoy!

In my family, we love eating this as a breakfast cereal with almond milk and fresh berries. My hubby loves it as a snack (I've had to hide stashes because otherwise he'll eat the whole batch within 24 hours). It's also used as a crunchy component in the Easy Autumn Parfait (page 327).

CHOCOLATE-ALMOND DIP

This is our version of Nutella. My kids love this spread on their toast for a snack or as a dip for fresh berries, apples, and even pineapple! I use almonds instead of the traditional hazelnuts because I buy them in bulk and use them more frequently in my cooking than I use hazelnuts, so I always have them on hand.

MAKES 2 CUPS (EIGHT ¼-CUP SERVINGS)

½ cup raw almonds
¼ cup unsweetened almond milk
⅔ cup pitted Medjool dates (about 6)
1 tablespoon unsweetened cocoa powder
½ teaspoon vanilla powder or vanilla extract, or seeds from 1 vanilla bean

Combine all the ingredients in a high-speed blender and blend on high until smooth and creamy, 60 to 90 seconds.

Storage: Store in the fridge in a glass food storage container or glass jar with a tight-fitting lid for up to 10 days.

CLASSIC VANILLA NICE CREAM

You can make legit-delicious ice cream with just fruit! This simple recipe was one of the biggest revelations on my whole-food plant-based journey. I've enjoyed this "nice cream" for so many years now that I actually prefer it to store-bought vegan ice cream, which tastes too sweet to me now. It's a great way to reduce commercial packaging, too.

MAKES 2 SERVINGS

2 tablespoons walnuts (optional, for richness)
4 large, extra-spotty bananas, peeled, sliced, and frozen at least overnight (see Note)
¼ teaspoon vanilla powder or vanilla extract (optional)
1 to 2 tablespoons unsweetened vanilla almond milk

Place the walnuts (if using) in a high-speed blender (see Note), then add the frozen bananas, the vanilla (if using), and finally 1 tablespoon of the almond milk. Blend until the bananas break down into a creamy, soft-serve-like consistency. The blending time may vary depending on your bananas but is generally around 30 seconds. To get things going, you'll really need to use the tamper for the first 20 seconds or so to help push down the banana slices into the blades. Just when you're convinced nothing is going to happen, the mixture will become creamy. Serve immediately.

Enjoy!

This nice cream is a huge deal at my house! My kids like theirs topped with Fridge Jam (page 253), a drizzle of raw almond butter, or coconut flakes.

Notes:

- Don't ditch those overly ripe bananas! For nice cream, the spottier and browner the banana peels, the better. I like to keep bananas on hand in a silicone storage bag in the freezer, where they'll keep for up to 3 months, but at a minimum, freeze the bananas overnight before making this recipe.
- As a banana ripens, its nutritional content shifts. The resistant starch in unripe bananas is transformed into sugars as the bananas turn yellow. Spotty bananas are the highest in sugars, and that's why they're frequently used in sweet recipes.
- You really want a powerful blender with a compact base (4 inches or less) for this recipe.

VEGGIE SCRAP BROTH

For a long time, I'd just toss all my veggie scraps into the compost. I figured that was definitely preferable to sending them to the landfill, but then I started developing a vegan pho recipe for my website and found out just how easy it is to make homemade broths using the scraps I would normally just toss out. When I prep and cook veggies, I store any scraps in plastic bins in the freezer, and once I've accumulated about 6 to 8 cups, I use them to make broth. I typically separate the scraps into three categories:

1. **Traditional:** carrot peels, yellow and white onions (peels, trimmed roots and tops, leftover pieces), celery stalks
2. **Asian:** mushrooms/mushroom stems; green, yellow, and white onions (peels, trimmed roots and tops, leftover pieces); celery; garlic; green cabbage; leek; ginger
3. **Red:** beets (peels and trimmings), red cabbage, red onion (peels, trimmed roots and tops, leftover pieces), red chard

Now I get three uses out of my veggies: eating the good parts, saving the scraps to make tasty broth, and composting the scraps after cooking the broth. I call that a win-win-win!

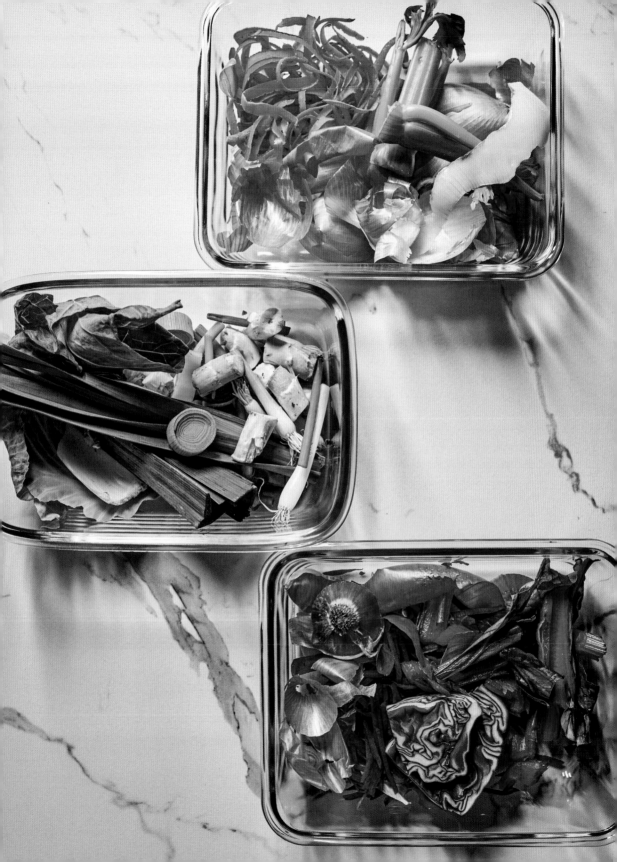

TRADITIONAL VEGGIE SCRAP BROTH

MAKES 12 TO 16 CUPS

6 to 8 cups vegetable scraps (see page 312 for preferred veggies)
1 large yellow onion, skin-on, halved
4 garlic cloves, peeled
1 to 2 teaspoons salt
1 or 2 bay leaves
1½ teaspoons olive oil (optional)

Put the vegetable scraps in a large stockpot and add water to cover. Add the onion, garlic, salt, bay leaf, and olive oil (if using).

Bring to a boil, then reduce the heat to medium-low and simmer for about 1 hour. Remove from the heat and let cool completely, then stir to mix well.

Stack a fine-mesh sieve over a widemouthed funnel and set them on top of a 1-quart glass jar. Strain the broth directly into the jar (you'll need three or four jars to hold all the broth); compost the solids. Let cool completely before storing.

Storage: Store in the fridge in glass jars with tight-fitting lids for up to 14 days. This broth freezes very well for up to 3 months; freeze in glass food storage containers (remember to leave 1 inch of headspace at the top of each), or freeze into cubes, then transfer to a silicone storage bag and store in the freezer.

Red Veggie Scrap Broth: I recommend keeping red veggie scraps out of your traditional broth and instead using them to make a beautiful red-hued broth. Just follow the same technique as for traditional broth using the veggies listed on page 312. I like using this red broth as a replacement for the water called for in Thai Curry Beet Soup (page 238). I also enjoy topping a bowl of red broth with chopped beet greens and green onions for a quick, warming, and highly nourishing soup.

ASIAN VEGGIE SCRAP BROTH

MAKES 8 TO 12 CUPS

4 to 6 cups vegetable scraps (see page 312 for preferred veggies)

1 large yellow onion, skin-on, halved

4 garlic cloves, peeled

1 knob ginger, peeled and cut into large dice

1 ounce dried shiitake mushrooms

1 lemongrass stalk, cut crosswise into 4 pieces

2 tablespoons white miso paste

2 tablespoons tamari

½ tablespoon sesame oil (optional)

Put the vegetable scraps in a large stockpot and add water to cover. Add the onion, garlic, ginger, mushrooms, lemongrass, miso, tamari, and sesame oil (if using).

Bring to a boil, then reduce the heat to medium-low and simmer for about 1 hour. Remove from the heat and let cool completely, then stir to mix well.

Stack a fine-mesh sieve over a widemouthed funnel and set them on top of a 1-quart glass jar. Strain the broth directly into the jar (you'll need two or three jars to hold all the broth); compost the solids (see Note). Let cool completely before storing.

Storage: Store in the fridge in glass jars with tight-fitting lids for up to 14 days. This broth freezes very well for up to 3 months; freeze in glass food storage containers (remember to leave 1 inch of headspace at the top of each), or freeze into cubes, then transfer to a silicone storage bag and store in the freezer.

Enjoy!

My favorite way to enjoy this broth is to make a vegan pho bowl with cooked noodles or raw zoodles and all the green veggies! My favorites are broccoli, zucchini, spinach, and even microgreens. The beauty is that you just add the raw veggies right to the hot broth, and it will lightly cook everything beautifully. When it's particularly cold outside, I'll eat this instead of a large salad to get all my greens in for the day!

Note: Sometimes I'll pick out the rehydrated shiitake mushrooms to serve with the broth instead of composting them; they'll keep in the fridge in a glass food storage container for up to 9 days.

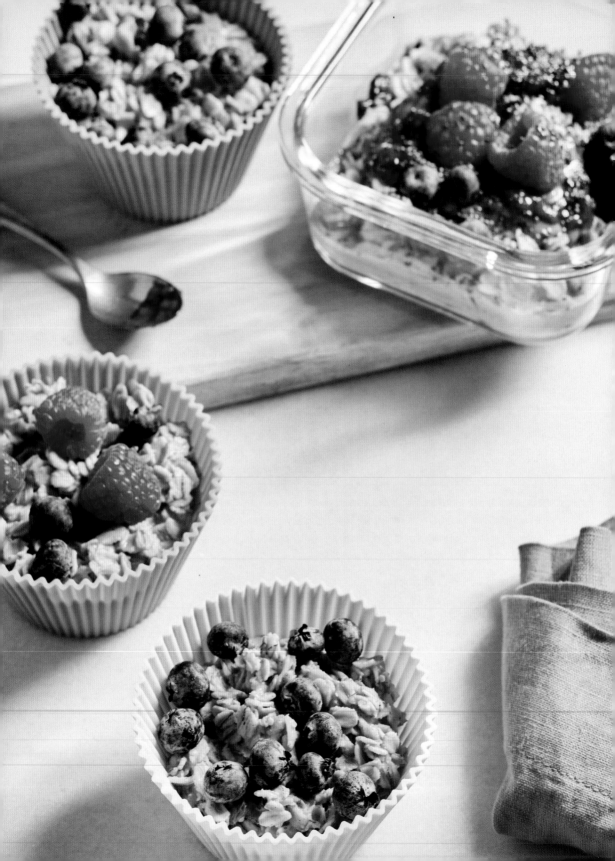

ON-DEMAND FAVORITES

The way to get the most out of your weekly prepping practice is to learn how to reconfigure components you've prepped ahead into easy-to-assemble on-demand meals. These are recipes you can make using prepped recipe components like sauces, dressings, and plant proteins. They can help you get a variety of meals from items you've already prepped, but they are designed to taste best when they're made to order!

LOADED OATMEAL BOWLS

My kids are huge breakfast lovers. On Saturdays, we make a big family brunch with both traditional and veganized breakfast classics—then on Sunday, we're back to our family oatmeal game! In the warmer months, that's usually overnight oats, but during the cooler, cozy months I'll make a big double batch of fresh, creamy oatmeal and arrange an oatmeal "bar" with all sorts of bits and bobs—leftover Fridge Jams, fresh and dried fruits, and nuts and seeds—for the whole family to share. This recipe is how I like to load up my personal bowl of oatmeal, but feel free to adjust the toppings to your liking and scale up the quantities to make more than one serving. When we're done with our Sunday-morning oats, the kids help me make Oatmeal Freezer Bowls (page 318) with the leftover cooked oatmeal. These freezer-friendly bowls are super-easy for the kids to heat up for themselves during the week. I just love this little two-in-one on-demand-and-prepping duo!

MAKES 1 SERVING

½ to 1 cup warm cooked rolled or steel-cut oats (cooked according to the package instructions)

½ to 1 tablespoon flaxseeds or hulled hemp seeds, or a mix

⅛ teaspoon vanilla powder (optional)

½ teaspoon ground cinnamon

1 to 2 tablespoons dried fruit (optional)

1 to 2 tablespoons runny unsalted nut butter (such as peanut or raw creamy almond)

¼ to ½ cup Blueberry Fridge Jam (page 257) or Raspberry Fridge Jam (page 257)

½ to 1 cup (chopped, if needed) fresh and/or frozen fruit (berries and apples work well)

1 teaspoon chia seeds, for garnish (optional)

Place the cooked oats in your bowl and add the flaxseeds, vanilla, ¼ teaspoon of the cinnamon, and the dried fruit (if using). Stir to combine well.

Top the oatmeal with the nut butter, jam, fruit, and chia seeds (if using), then sprinkle with the remaining ¼ teaspoon cinnamon.

Storage: Store leftovers in the fridge in a glass food storage container with a tight-fitting lid for 3 to 4 days.

Oatmeal Freezer Bowls

YIELD VARIES

Cooked oatmeal (you can use leftovers from Loaded Oatmeal Bowls, page 317)
Maple syrup
Optional add-ins: berries, chopped fresh or frozen fruit, raisins, flaxseeds, nut butter, seeds, coconut

Put the oatmeal in a small bowl and stir in a little maple syrup. Stir in the add-ins of your choice, reserving some for topping. Transfer the mixture to a silicone baking cup, filling it about three-quarters full, then top with the reserved add-ins (this will help you easily identify what flavor the oatmeal cups are). Set the cups on a baking sheet and freeze overnight.

Turn the frozen oatmeal cups out of the molds and transfer them to a plastic freezer container or silicone storage bag.

Storage: Store in the freezer for up to 2 months (with two kids, these tend to go quickly in our home!). To reheat, place in microwave-safe bowl and microwave on high for 2 to 3 minutes.

QUICK AND CRISPY ITALIAN HUMMUS FLATBREAD PIZZA

Pizza cravings happen, and when they do, I like to be prepared with a healthy option that assuages that urge with the healthiest options possible. Enter this hummus flatbread "pizza"!

MAKES 1 SERVING

1 pita bread
3 to 4 tablespoons your favorite marinara sauce
¼ cup Italian Herb Cannellini Bean Hummus (page 185; see Note)
Classic Vegan Parmesan (page 190; optional)
Chopped fresh herbs, such as parsley and basil, for garnish (optional)

Preheat the oven to 375°F. Line a baking sheet with parchment paper or a silicone baking mat.

Spread the marinara sauce evenly over the pita bread. Top with dollops of the hummus and sprinkle with parmesan (if using). Place the pita on the prepared baking sheet.

Bake for 15 to 20 minutes, rotating the pan once halfway through, until the pita is just crispy and the hummus is beginning to brown around the edges.

Garnish with fresh herbs, if desired.

Note: You can replace the hummus with store-bought plant-based almond-milk ricotta cheese (Kite Hill is an excellent brand) and add a sprinkling of vegan or dairy mozzarella cheese.

QUICK AND CRISPY SPINACH AND ARTICHOKE FLATBREAD

I love how quickly flatbreads come together if you've already prepped your sauces and dips for the week. I try to pick up a package of pita bread at the store every couple of weeks (they keep for up to 2 weeks in the fridge) so I can make these flatbreads when the craving strikes. I like to serve them with a cup of soup or salad.

MAKES 1 SERVING

1 pita bread
⅓ to ½ cup unbaked Spinach and Artichoke Dip (page 242)
Pickled red onion (see page 198), for topping (optional)
¼ teaspoon raw sesame seeds, for garnish (optional)

Preheat the oven to 375°F. Line a baking sheet with parchment paper or a silicone baking mat.

Spread the spinach and artichoke dip evenly over the pita bread. Top with the pickled onions and/or sesame seeds (if using). Place the pita on the prepared baking sheet.

Bake for 15 to 20 minutes, rotating the pan once halfway through, until the pita is just crispy and the dip is just beginning to brown around the edges.

Note: If desired, you can sprinkle the flatbread with your favorite vegan or dairy cheese before baking or add a drizzle of olive oil before or after baking.

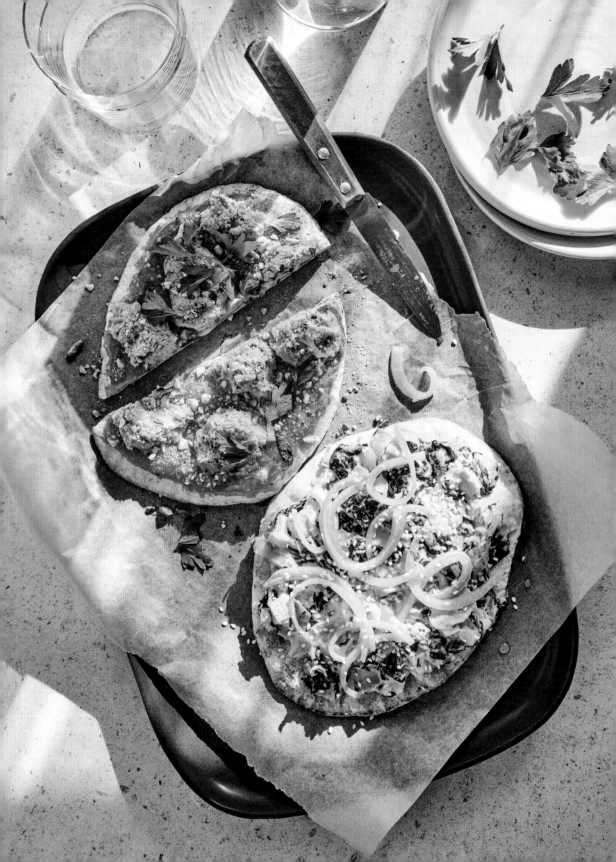

RAINBOW COLLARD WRAPS

Sometimes a girl just can't eat another salad—sorry (not sorry!). On those days, these wraps are a good alternative. Collard leaves, which are amazingly nutritious, make the most amazing natural wrappers!

MAKES 1 SERVING

3 large collard green leaves (6 inches wide or larger)
½ avocado
1 teaspoon lime juice
1⅓ cups shredded or very thinly sliced (on a mandoline) rainbow veggies, such as beets, carrots (orange and yellow), red bell pepper, and red cabbage
⅓ cup Peanut Coconut Sauce (page 171) or Sweet-and-Sour Sauce (page 191), for dipping

Trim off the stems of the collard leaves at the base of each leaf, then use a vegetable peeler to shave down the protruding center rib on the back side of the leaves. Wash the leaves.

Place one collard leaf at a time on a microwave-safe plate and microwave for 10 to 15 seconds. The leaf will turn bright green and become more pliable. Set aside on a plate and repeat with the remaining collards.

Mash the avocado in a small bowl. Add the lime juice and mix well.

Position a collard leaf on a cutting board with the center rib running horizontally, parallel to you. Spread one-third of the avocado mixture in the middle of the leaf just below the center rib. Pile a third of the shredded veggies on top of the avocado. Fold the lower half of the leaf over the filling and tuck in the filling using your fingers, tightly packing the filling so it doesn't come out when cutting the wraps. Fold in the sides toward the filling and roll the wrap up away from you. Repeat with the remaining leaves and filling.

Use a serrated knife to slice each roll in half on an angle. Serve with your desired dipping sauce.

Note: To make these a heartier meal, you could also add some cooked rice noodles and sliced strips of Easy Baked Tofu (page 271).

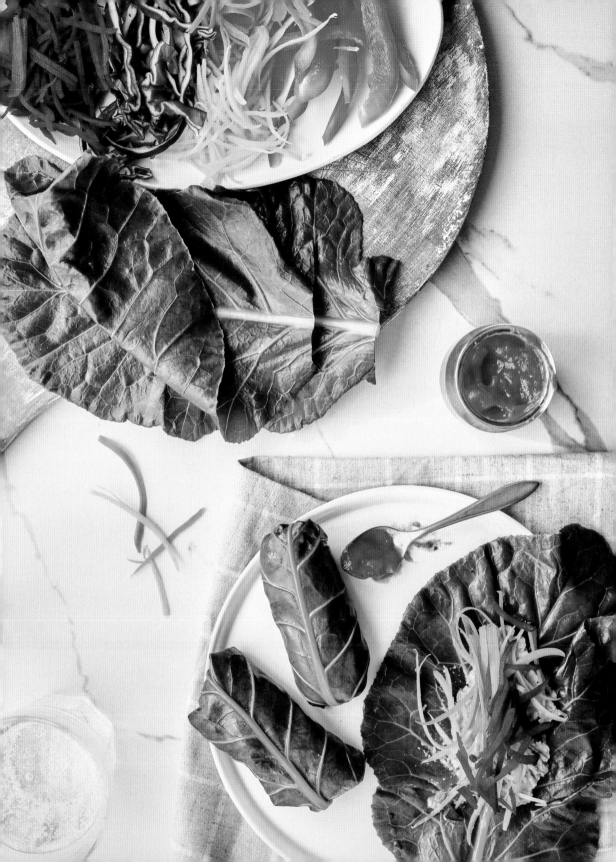

EASY TACO SLIDERS

About a year ago, I found the cutest mini corn tortillas, about 3½ inches in diameter, at the store. I'm not one to be able to resist cute little things, so I grabbed a pack for our weekly Taco Tuesdays. We quickly realized that the best part about eating mini tacos is that you get to eat A LOT of tacos! These are perfectly kid-size and would also make a great appetizer or snack for a party.

MAKES 10 MINI TACOS (TWO 5-TACO SERVINGS)

3 tablespoons mayo, homemade (page 192) or store-bought (vegan or conventional)
2 teaspoons lime juice or distilled white vinegar
2 cups shredded red or green cabbage, or a mix
2 tablespoons fresh cilantro leaves (optional, but recommended)
10 small (3½-inch) corn tortillas (such as Mi Rancho brand)
½ cup plus 2 tablespoons canned black beans, drained and rinsed
5 tablespoons Nacho Cheese Sauce (page 188)
1 recipe Tofu Taco Meat (page 273)
Fresh Pico de Gallo (page 193) or your favorite hot sauce or salsa, for serving

In a medium bowl, whisk together the mayo and lime juice. Add the cabbage and cilantro (if using) and toss well. Set aside.

Warm the tortillas in the microwave for 20 to 30 seconds or in a preheated 350°F oven for about 5 minutes. If desired, warm the beans.

Spread the tortillas with the cheese sauce, then top evenly with the tofu taco meat, beans, and cabbage mixture. Top with pico de gallo or your favorite hot sauce or salsa. Serve immediately!

NUTTY BANANA SMOOTHIE

A few years ago, I joined a CrossFit gym when one of my best friends begged me to do it with her. I almost passed out a few times that first week and I haven't been back since our trial membership expired, but I will say that one very amazing thing came from that experience: the creation of this smoothie! I'd literally fantasize about getting home to this smoothie, which I used as my "reward" for the burpees, planks, and bear crawls I endured. It single-handedly got me through that month of, well, torture! Now my whole family—and my friend Lisa—enjoys this as a dessert or an extra-special after-workout treat!

MAKES 1 SMOOTHIE (ABOUT 2 CUPS)

1 cup sliced frozen bananas

3 raw walnut halves

1 tablespoon ground flaxseed

¼ cup rolled oats

1 tablespoon almond butter

½ teaspoon ground cinnamon

1¼ cups unsweetened almond milk

1 or 2 Medjool dates, pitted and chopped

Combine all the ingredients in a high-speed blender. Blend on high for 30 seconds, or until smooth and creamy.

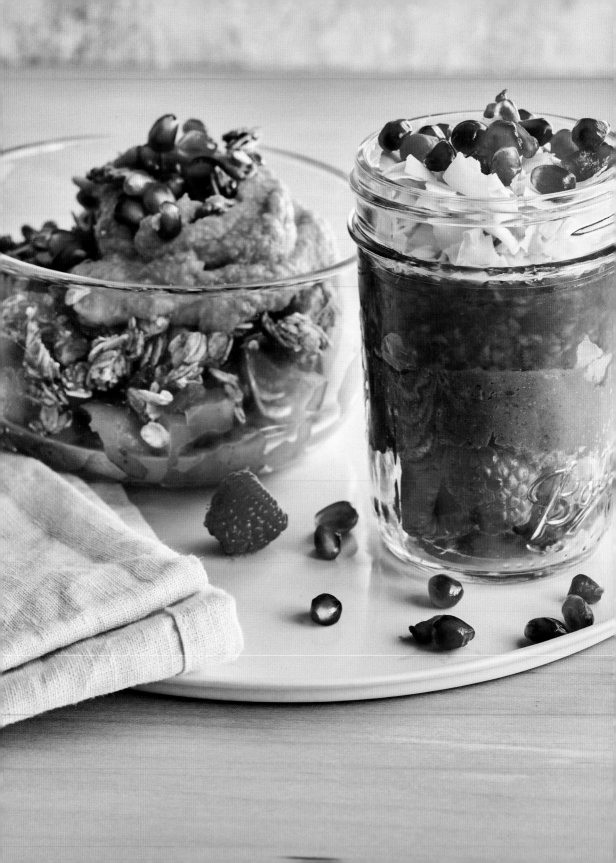

ALWAYS EASY PARFAITS

These are two of my favorite desserts! Using sweet hummus in these recipes is a smart health hack, since the soluble fiber in the hummus naturally limits your body's insulin response to high-glycemic foods. These parfaits make me feel special while taming my sweet tooth in a responsible, nontriggering way!

EASY CHOCOLATE PARFAIT

MAKES 1 PARFAIT

¼ cup Raspberry Fridge Jam
(page 257)
¼ cup Chocolate Hummus (page 187)
¼ cup fresh raspberries
1 to 2 tablespoons pomegranate seeds,
for garnish (optional)
Unsweetened flaked or shredded coconut, for garnish (optional)

In a dessert glass, cup, or jar, layer the jam, hummus, and raspberries. Sprinkle with the pomegranate seeds and coconut, if desired. Serve immediately.

EASY AUTUMN PARFAIT

MAKES 1 PARFAIT

¼ cup Cinnamon-Apple Fridge Jam
(page 256)
½ cup Oil-Free Fruit-Sweetened Nut or
Seed Granola (page 308)
¼ cup Pumpkin Hummus (page 186)
1 to 2 tablespoons pomegranate seeds,
for topping (optional)

In a dessert glass or cup, layer the jam, most of the granola, and the hummus. Sprinkle with the pomegranate seeds, if desired, and top with the remaining granola. Serve immediately.

ACKNOWLEDGMENTS

I signed the contract for this book exactly one month before the world changed forever. I could not have juggled two kids' remote learning, a home business, and a project of this magnitude without the flexibility afforded to me by HarperCollins*Publishers* and my amazing editor, Stephanie Fletcher. Thank you for your incredible belief in this project and your craftsmanship in making this the best possible resource it could be!

To my lovely agent, Michele Crim, for making that trip to the second coffee shop and ultimately taking a chance on my vision for a very different kind of cookbook.

Kevin, thank you for guarding my dreams as closely as your own. Thank you for the late-night pep talks, for jumping in whenever I needed you, for the endless rounds of dirty dishes, and your perfectly-cooked 3 AM falafel.

To my children, Kysen and Kamryn, you are always my inspiration to try the scary things and to push myself farther than feels comfortable.

To my father, Robert, for taking the time to watch the Dr. Fuhrman PBS special that changed our lives forever. To my mother, Marianne, my sister, Suzie, and my aunt, Marilyn, for all the advice, encouragement and California-Florida phone calls we shared as I worked on this project.

To my best friend, Lisa, who convinced me to go for this dream. Thank you for the check-in texts, late-night chats and relentless enthusiasm throughout this project. Tag, you're it!

To Amy, for helping me test and develop these recipes—I'm so grateful to have you as my work-sister! To Jenn, for helping me feel comfortable both in front of and behind the camera. To Priscilla, for helping me feel confident during every major moment in my career with your honest words and beautiful work.

To the people who have always been kind enough to let me know that they believed in what I was doing: Soo, Minna, Julie, Lisa H., Amanda, Jenna, Suzanne, Kelly, Gail, Carrie, Bethany, and Courtney.

And finally, to my entire Hello Nutritarian community for your love and support throughout the years.

INDEX